VICTORIAN GROTESQUE

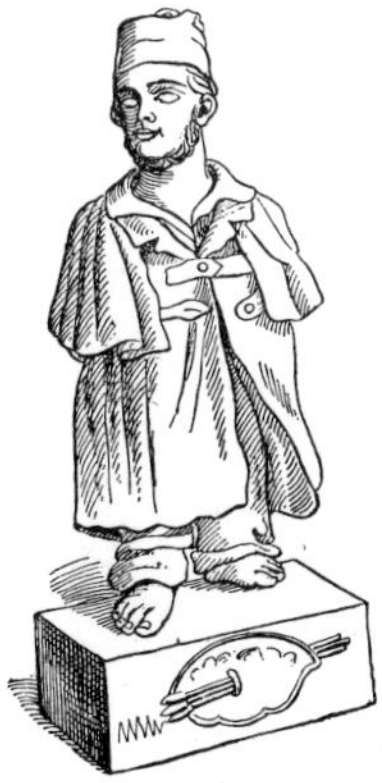

VICTORIAN GROTESQUE

AN ILLUSTRATED EXCURSION INTO
MEDICAL CURIOSITIES, FREAKS AND ABNORMALITIES –
PRINCIPALLY OF THE VICTORIAN AGE

by MARTIN HOWARD

LONDON
JUPITER BOOKS
1977

First published in 1977 by
JUPITER BOOKS (LONDON) LIMITED
167 Hermitage Road, London N4 1LZ

SBN 904041 75 1

Composed in 12-point Monotype Old Style, Series 2,
and printed and bound in Great Britain
by R. J. Acford Limited, Industrial Estate, Chichester, Sussex

CONTENTS

1 A TALENT FOR THE BIZARRE 11

2 INCIDENCE OF MAJOR TERATA 21

3 DESPERATE BUT NOT SERIOUS 43

4 GIANTS, DWARFS, FAT LADIES AND LIVING SKELETONS 93

5 HUMAN SMELLS, ADDICTIONS, EXTRAORDINARY FEATS 123

6 STRANGE CUSTOMS, STRANGER MISFORTUNES . . 147

VICTORIAN GROTESQUE

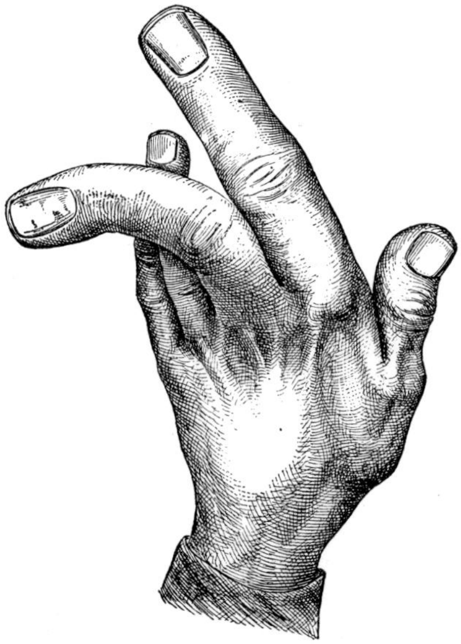

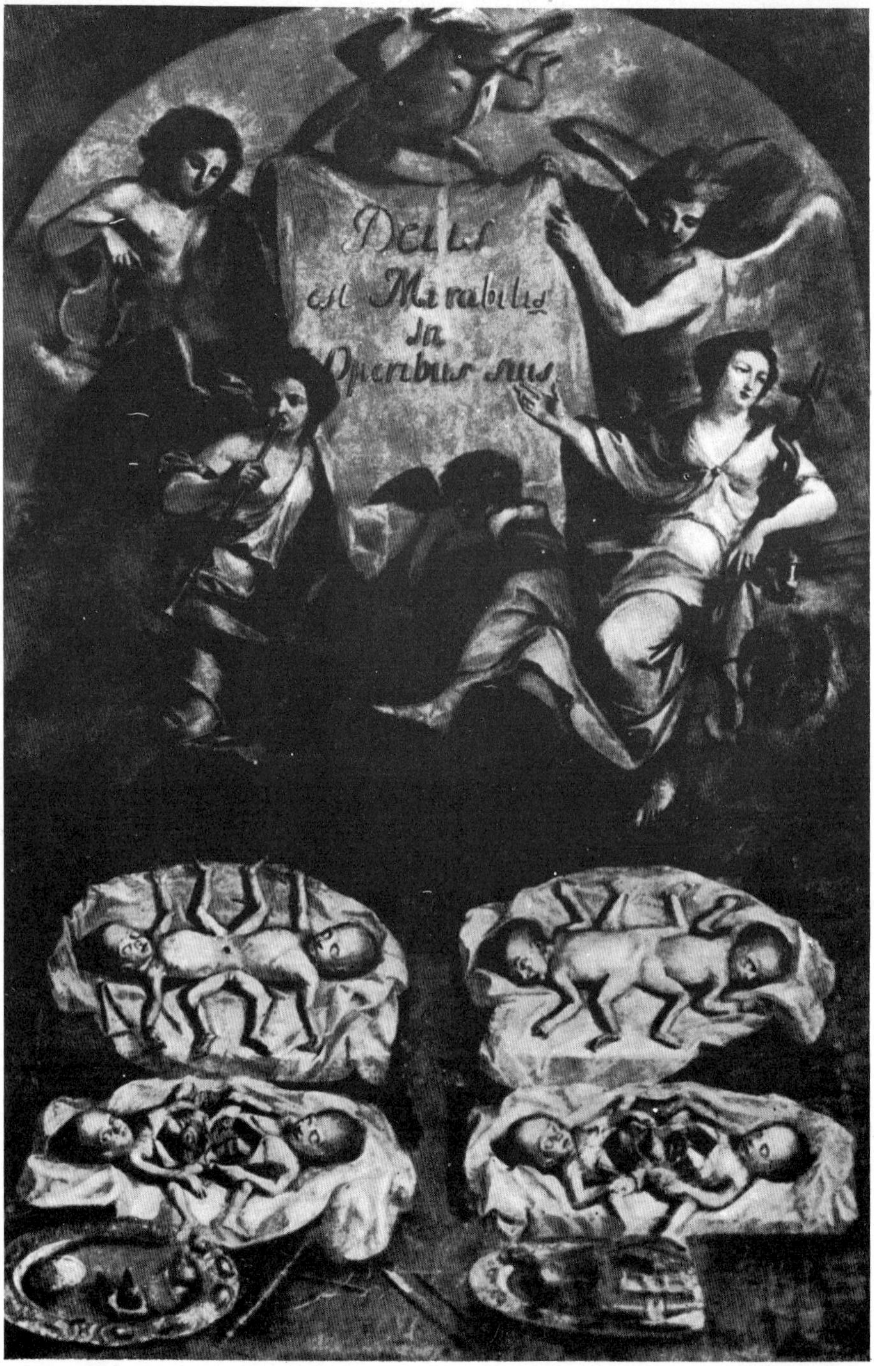

An engraving by Nicolas Sauvage, 1704, in commemoration of the dissection of Siamese twins by Johannès Palfyn: *God is Marvellous in All His Works*.

CHAPTER ONE

A TALENT FOR THE BIZARRE

TERATOLOGY, a word meaning 'tales of the marvellous', has been pinched by the scientists to refer to the study of monstrosities. Terata are monstrous formations or births. Monsters are not frightening. They are marvels, prodigies, sent by the gods as omens and as treasuries of fresh information. As the accompanying proclamation reads, commemorating a dissection of Siamese twins in 1704, *God is Marvellous in All His Works*. ¶ Monsters are deviants from normal development. People are frankly interested in deviants today. In Victorian times they had to be deviously interested. You were allowed to be interested in science so long as you quickly turned over the pages that would shock 'the man on the Clapham omnibus'. Now, the man on the Clapham omnibus is looking over your shoulder. ¶ The Victorian period was the great age for detailed and reliable research into teratology, the culmination of which was found in George Gould and Walter Pyle's *Anomalies and Curiosities of Medicine* (1896), a massive crown quarto volume of very nearly a thousand pages. The foundations of the scientific study had been laid earlier, in the eighteenth century. Before that time the only account in which reasonable trust could be reposed was the painstaking effort of Ambroise Paré, whose collected works were printed in Paris in 1598. Albrecht von Haller, writing in Switzerland but using the Latin language, produced between 1746 and 1774 a body of work which included *Bibliotheca anatomica*, *Bibliotheca chirurgica*, and *Elementa physiologiae corporis humani sensibilibus et irritabilibus*. Although he had trained as a doctor at Tübingen and Leyden, his first burst was into poetry, using the German language and dynamically revivifying it. He was professor of anatomy, botany, and medicine at Göttingen between 1736 and 1753, and then retired to Berne to produce his exhaustive commentaries of medical knowledge, the most relevant of which is *De Monstris*. At the same time Régnault was completing his *Recueil des principales monstruosités que la nature produit dans le monde animal*. In Padua Giovanni Battista Morgagni, professor of anatomy at the university there for fifty-six years, established pathological anatomy as a science with his *De sedibus et causis morborum*. ¶ The specialized pursuit of teratology was taken up by French writers in a great explosion of energy that coincided with the reign of Queen Victoria. The father and son team of Étienne and Isidore Geoffroy Saint-Hilaire consummated their work, and celebrated the Queen's accession, with Isidore's *Histoire des anomalies de l'organisation chez l'homme et les animaux*, and his *Traité de Tératologie*. F. E. Guérin published an illustrated dictionary of phenomena, Lancereaux an atlas of pathological anatomy; Jules Guérin issued his researches on deformities, and Martin his history of monsters. Guinard published his *Précis de Tératologie* in 1893, and the era was crowned with Camille Dareste's curious work, *Recherches sur la production artificielle des monstruosités*. Alongside this commentary in depth, the medical journals applied themselves to the subject whenever their case histories offered. This present work has sprung from research among 720 Victorian manuals and medical reviews in general, and the work of Gould and Pyle, already mentioned, in particular. ¶ Victorian interest in the grotesque was reflected in the public reception of teratology. This was the age of Phineas T. Barnum, as well as of the queen who was not amused. She was amused, in point of fact, by one of Barnum's greatest showbiz creations, General Tom Thumb – an amiable dwarf who captured the affections of many monarchs and presidents, and, naturally, of less blue-blooded members of High Society. Cora Pearl, the Cockney courtesan who became the richly rewarded mistress of the brother of the Emperor Napoleon III, conceived the idea of sleeping with Tom Thumb for a kick. She was famous for appearing at her own dinner parties as the entrée of the evening, on a huge silver salver carried in by four footmen who whisked off the silver cover and exposed her naked. But this time it was Tom Thumb whom she conveyed to her boudoir, delicately poised in one hand on a silver dish no bigger than that used for the Christmas turkey. Barnum made an honest man of Tom Thumb after that scandal by personally supervising his marriage to Lavinia Warren, a little lady of about Tom's own stature whom Barnum had brought back from England. England had fallen in such a big way for Tom Thumb, and Tom Thumb had fallen so deeply for the English, that the dwarf kissed every Englishwoman he met. It was said – by Barnum, naturally – that altogether Tom Thumb had kissed one million Englishwomen, but not Queen Victoria, to whom he was presented in 1844 (he was only twelve years old then). ¶ The great Tom Thumb wedding, masterminded by Barnum in 1864, was put on as a diversion from – though some observers say as the climax of – the horrors of the American Civil War. Those who belong to the latter school of thought are perhaps unduly influenced by the marital careers of the original 'Siamese' twins, Eng and Chang, who had also married Englishwomen and returned to the United States. Eng and Chang had originally fled from America, where they were put on show after their discovery in Siam, to escape the pursuit of a voracious show-business nymphomaniac named Miss

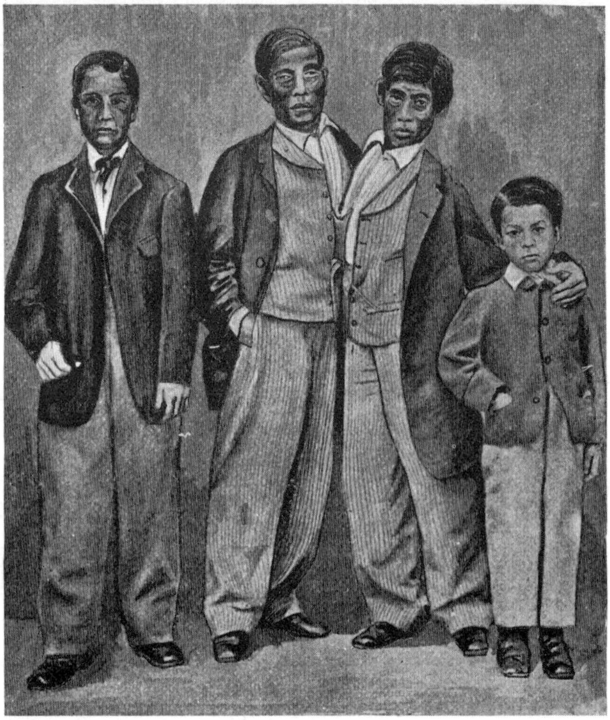

The original
Siamese Twins
in old age.

Gloria, who wanted to marry them both, and had published over-explicit erotic verses celebrating their twin charms. So when they were thirty-two, they married two sisters named Sarah and Adelaide Yates, aged twenty-six and twenty-eight, and settled down to farm in North Carolina. Unfortunately, however, the sisters fought each other so remorselessly that the twins had to set up two homes, some distance apart, and they would jog from one to the other on horseback. Each master bedroom naturally had to contain a bed for three. By skilful manipulation of this arrangement Chang and Eng fathered ten and twelve children respectively before they died within three hours of each other at the age of sixty-two. ¶ Another pair of Siamese twins, Lucio and Simplicio, married twin sisters and used to put on a great show dancing the tango together. They also graduated as champion ice-skaters. But they came to grief in a stormy drama. One of them got drunk and caused a carriage accident in which a child was run over. He was hauled

Rosa and Josepha Blazek. Rosa, on the right, holds her child.

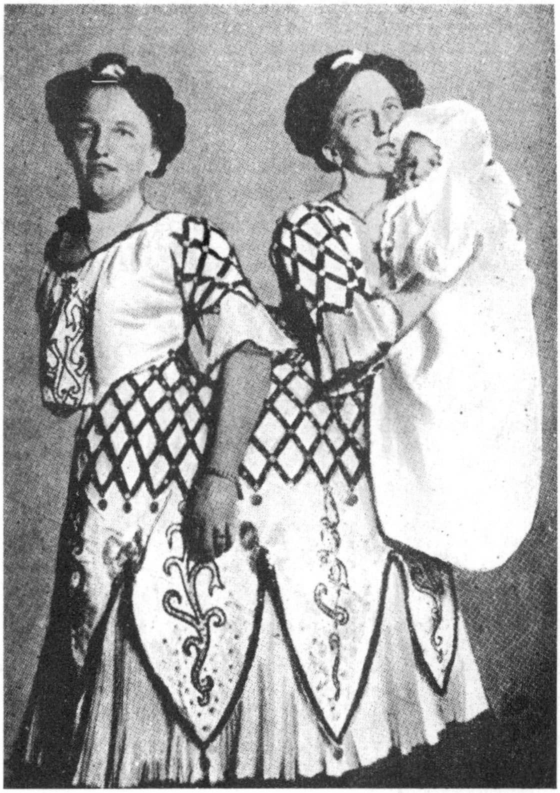

off to court, and naturally his brother had to go with him. The judge was forced to concede that he could not send the guilty party to prison without also punishing his innocent brother by confining him to the same cell. He therefore imposed a heavy fine which would have to be paid out of personal earnings. But the innocent brother, thoroughly fed up, declared that he was not going to exhibit himself with his partner just to pay the other's fine, and he had quite enough to live on as it was. So the guilty brother reacted by threatening to commit suicide, which would automatically end the other's life. ¶ Rosa and Josepha Blazek, a pair of Siamese twin sisters, got up to some hanky-panky and Rosa was delivered of a bouncing baby in Vienna. At the inevitable inquest sister Josepha declared that she hadn't seen a thing, and couldn't understand it. But their astute manager soon discovered the father, in the person of a

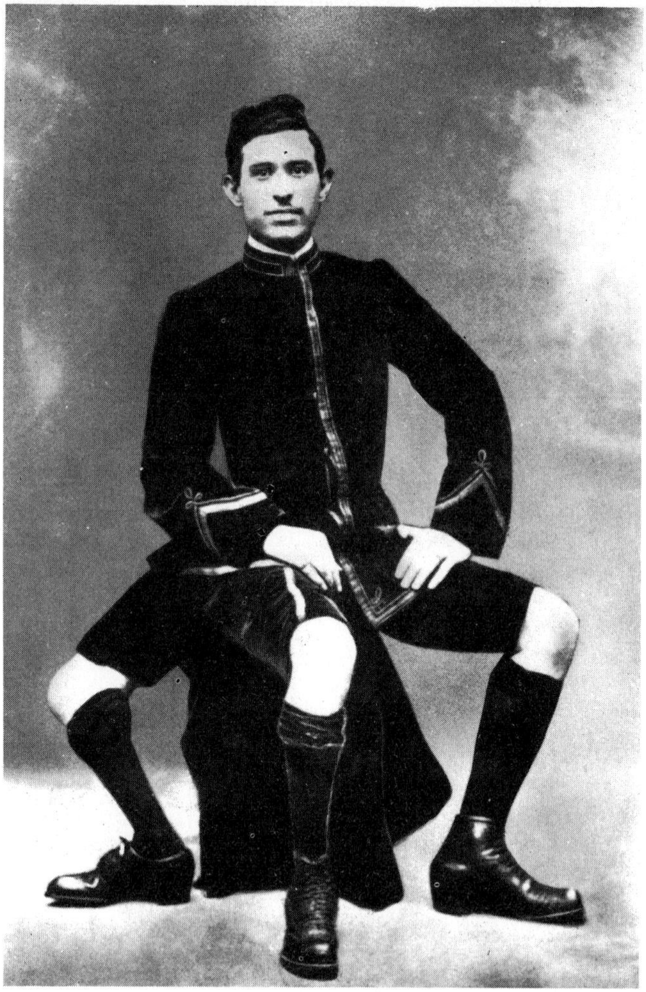

Francesco Lentini: the human tripod.

strapping butcher. Punishment? How could he do anything but condone such an understandable indiscretion? And make the best of it. He whisked the twins, the butcher, and the baby off to Paris, where the whole family went on show with overwhelming success at the Théâtre de la Gaîté. ¶ Francesco Lentini, a pygomelian with three legs who made a fortune by exhibiting himself in short trousers, found to his dismay that he had enflamed the passions of a wealthy lady from central Europe who kidnapped him in order that she could enjoy him exclusively. But Lentini got bored, escaped, and went on the exhibition circuit again.

Mme Delait, the most celebrated bearded woman. From a contemporary French postcard.

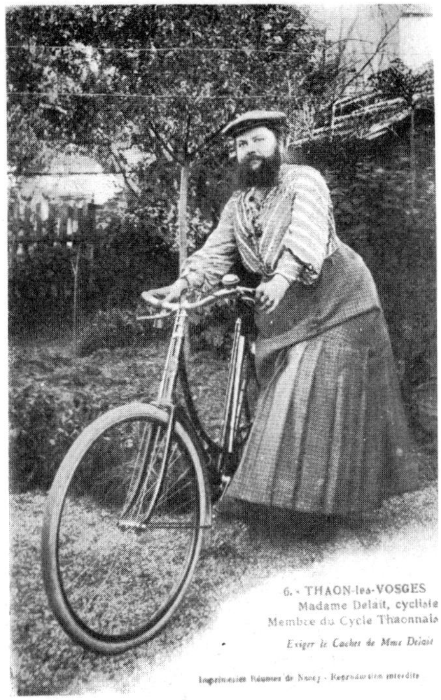
6. - THAON-les-VOSGES
Madame Delait, cycliste
Membre du Cycle Thaonnais
Exiger le Cachet de Mme Delait

A famous French bearded lady, Madame Delait, compromised with her beard to the extent that she wore trouser-skirts to go bicycling – a bold step in the old-fashioned milieu of the rural Vosges district, though the trousers were voluminous enough. Showman Barnum's bearded lady married the alligator-man who had been occupying the neighbouring caravan when they went on tour. ¶ But the height of Victorian Grotesque was reached in the memorable fate of Julia Pastrana, the gorilla-woman, known professionally as 'the Ugliest Woman in the World'. She was no artificially made-up circus freak: Charles Darwin examined her and recorded: 'This woman had a strong beard, a very hairy body, particularly on the forehead and the neck and, a phenomenon of particular interest, an irregular double row of teeth in the upper and lower jaw which gave her a prognathic appearance and a simian profile.' Julia Pastrana fell in love with her manager. His immediate reaction was that he did not wish to lose an exhibit which was bringing him a fortune; so he married her, and soon she was expecting a baby.

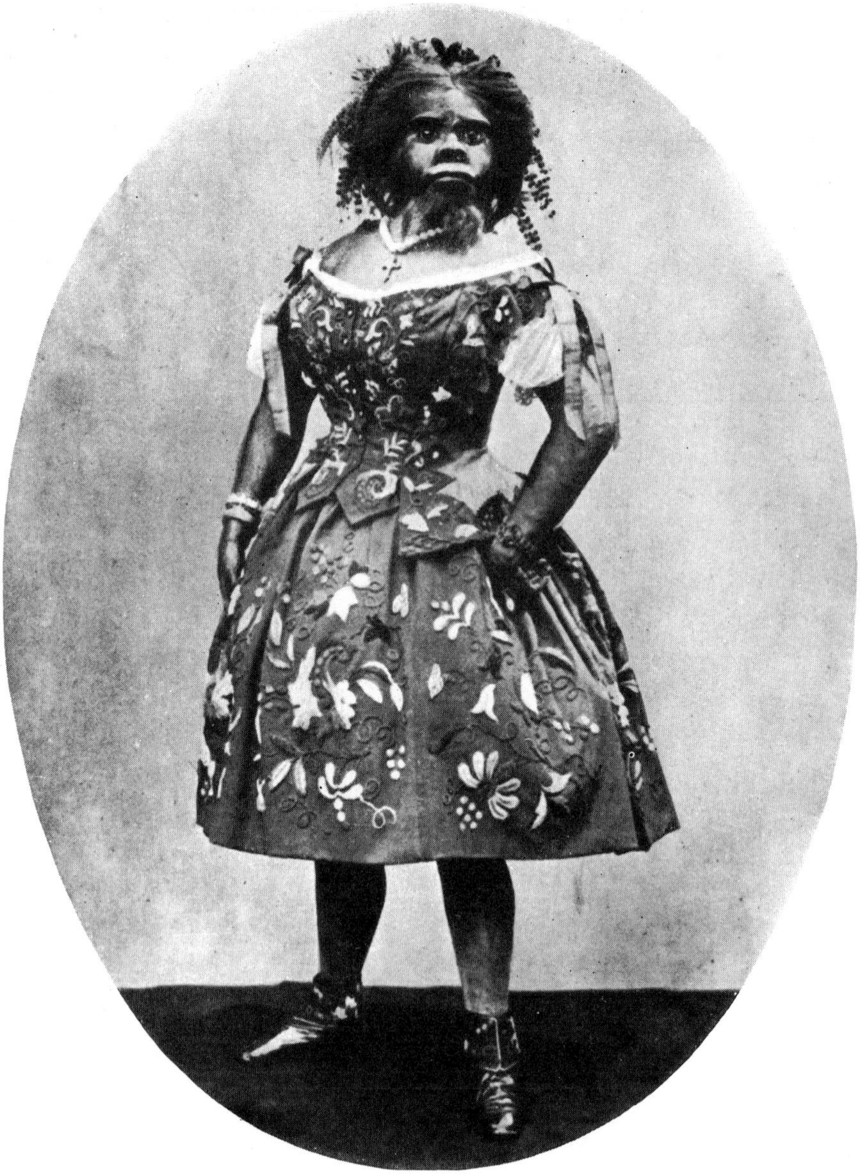

Julia Pastrana, the gorilla-woman.

Victorian society waited with bated breath to see what the result of this union would be. A throng of aristocrats and snobs flocked to the drawing room of the house which had been selected for the accouchement. The child was born, very hairy and physically doomed. Julia herself was in a very bad condition and soon it was clear that she too would die. Society filed by her bedside. Into the ear of a passing princess she whispered her own pathetic epitaph: 'I die happy, for I know that I have been loved for myself.' As soon as she was dead the manager-husband had both bodies stuffed by a taxidermist, and exhibited them all over Europe, clothed in shoddy stage tinsel and decked with artificial jewellery. ¶ Whatever could be said about the Victorians, their successors could at least raise a merrier laugh out of the grotesque. Little Tich, the famous tiny music-hall comedian, used to go out into the public parks dressed as a little boy, and tie himself into knots as he went through the motions (or almost went through the motions) of an innocent small lad who simply could not wait to spend a penny. Nursemaids used to take pity on him, and he responded by being so obviously clumsy, awkward, and helpless that they obligingly helped to unbutton him. The shrieks that followed enlivened the afternoon scene, though they occasionally led to appearances in the magistrate's court for outraging public decency.

RIGHT

A drawing, based on that of Galvagni, of a three-headed monster.

BELOW

Infant with a supernumary head.

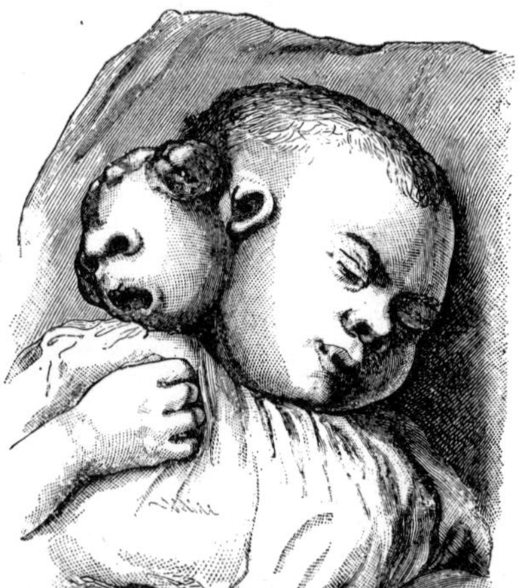

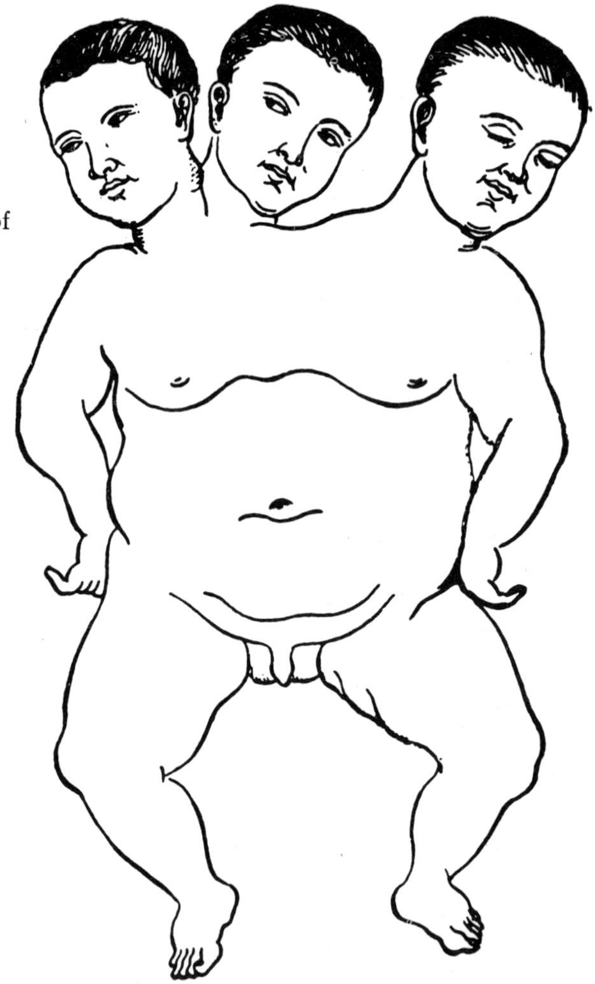

CHAPTER TWO

INCIDENCE OF MAJOR TERATA

MAJOR TERATA comprise the issue of those births which result from the union of more than one foetus or display the duplication of limbs or other members through abnormal cell-division in the embryo. The classic monster, and indeed the cliché monster, is the being with two heads – a condition which has been adopted so widely as a symbol of buffoon cretinism that it is frequently used by newspaper editors as a pleasantry to describe their average reader. On rare occasions humans have been born with three heads, and there is a fairly reliable drawing of one observed by Galvagni at Catania, Sicily, in 1834. Martin de Pedro described a similar case which occurred in Madrid in 1879. Sutton's *Clinical Sketches* of 1895 mentions a child seen in Bristol which had a supernumerary head with a conventionally shaped mouth and nose, but the eyes were shut and an ear was rudimentary. The nurse said that when the child sucked, some milk was regurgitated through the second mouth. When the natural face cried or yawned, the supernumerary

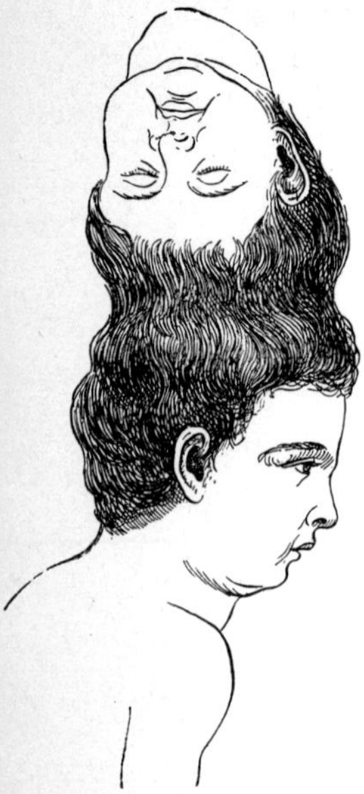

Two-headed boy.

face duplicated these movements exactly. The brain of the attached head was quite separate, and visible through a membrane. An earlier authenticated case was of a child born in Bengal with a supernumerary head reversed on its skull. Both heads functioned separately, and when one was given milk, the mouth of the other filled with saliva. The child died of snake-bite when it was four years old, and its skull was sent to the museum of the Royal College of Surgeons in London. There have been more modern instances of this phenomenon, one of which is a fusion of the bones of the cranium. ¶ The most pathetic instance of this abnormality was the case of Edward Mordake, said to have been heir to a noble family in England, of whom it is recounted: 'He lived in complete seclusion, refusing the visits even of members of his own family. He was a young man of fine attainments, a profound scholar, and a musician of rare ability. His figure was remarkable for its grace, and his face – that is to say, his natural face – was that of an Antinous. But upon the back of his head was another face, that of a beautiful girl, "lovely as a dream, hideous as a devil". The female face was a mere mask, "occupying only a small portion of the posterior part of the skull, yet exhibiting every sign of intelligence, of a malignant sort, however". It would be seen to smile and sneer while Mordake was weeping. The eyes would follow the movements of the spectator, and the lips would "gibber without ceasing". No voice was audible, but Mordake averred that he was kept from his rest at night by the hateful whispers of his "devil twin", as he called it, "which never sleeps, but talks to me forever of such things as they only speak of in hell. No imagination can conceive the dreadful temptations it sets before me. For some unforgiven wickedness of my forefathers I am knit to this fiend – for a fiend it surely is. I beg and beseech you to crush it out of human resemblance, even if I die for it". Such were the words of the hapless Mordake to Manvers and Treadwell, his physicians. In spite of careful watching he managed to procure poison, whereof he died, leaving a letter requesting that the "demon face" might be destroyed before

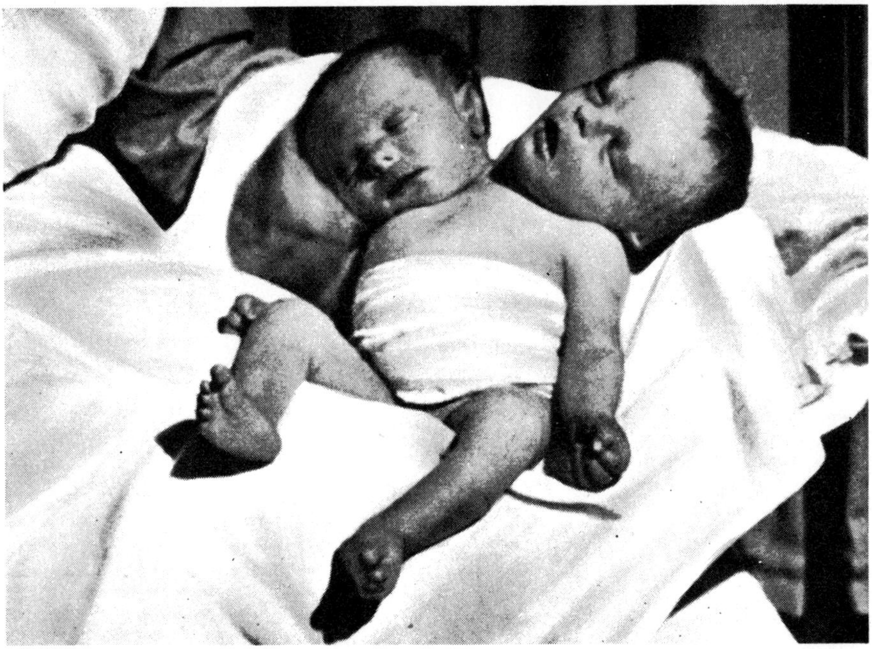

A child born with two heads; a photograph taken in a Paris hospital in the 1950s.

his burial, "lest it continues its dreadful whisperings even in my grave". At his own request he was interred in a waste place, without stone or legend to mark his grave.' ¶ Less like a story by Edgar Allan Poe was the more common union of two distinct foetuses which was apparent in Eng and Chang, the original 'Siamese' twins, who were born on 11 May 1811 at Maklong, Thailand, though their parents were Chinese. They were joined, as were others of their kind who were well known in Victorian times, by a cartilaginous band which extended from the sternum of one to that of the other by a union of the ensiform cartilages, that is, a joining of the sword-shaped prolongation at the bottom of the breast-bone of each. They were the fifth delivery of their mother, who afterwards had several sets of twins and in all bore fourteen children. The junction was over four inches long, and comparatively plastic, so that they were not compelled to live face to face, but usually walked with their arms about each other's farther shoulder. And for most of their long lives they did not hate each other as did Edward Mordake and his 'demon

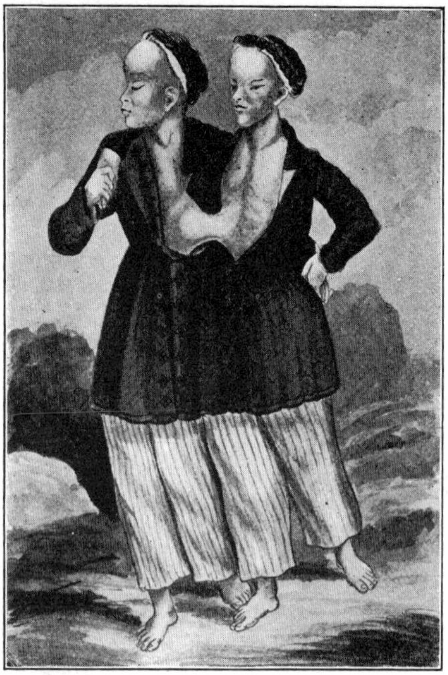

Chang and Eng, the Siamese Twins, at the age of eighteen years.

FACING

A contemporary print of the Twins in their youth.

face'. ¶ The twins were sickly at birth, though Chang emerged stronger than Eng. Their survival was not encouraged, since the reigning King of Siam, Chowpahyi, believed, as had many of the ancients, that the birth was a bad omen for himself and his country. But they were seen at Bangkok by a British merchant, Robert Hunter, who persuaded the king to let them leave the country, and then put them in the hands of a Captain Coffin to exploit them by exhibiting them. Coffin's name was another omen which did not come true. At the age of eight the twins arrived at Harvard University for a full professional medical examination, after which they went on an exhibition tour of the Eastern states of America. Afterwards they went on a number of tours in Europe, though their exhibition was prohibited in some countries in case the sight of them caused women spectators to produce similar children. After their marriage in America, and the necessary establishment of two homes which has been mentioned, they fell on bad times and resolved on another tour of Europe. The reason they gave was that they had had a particular quarrel, and from that moment had conceived

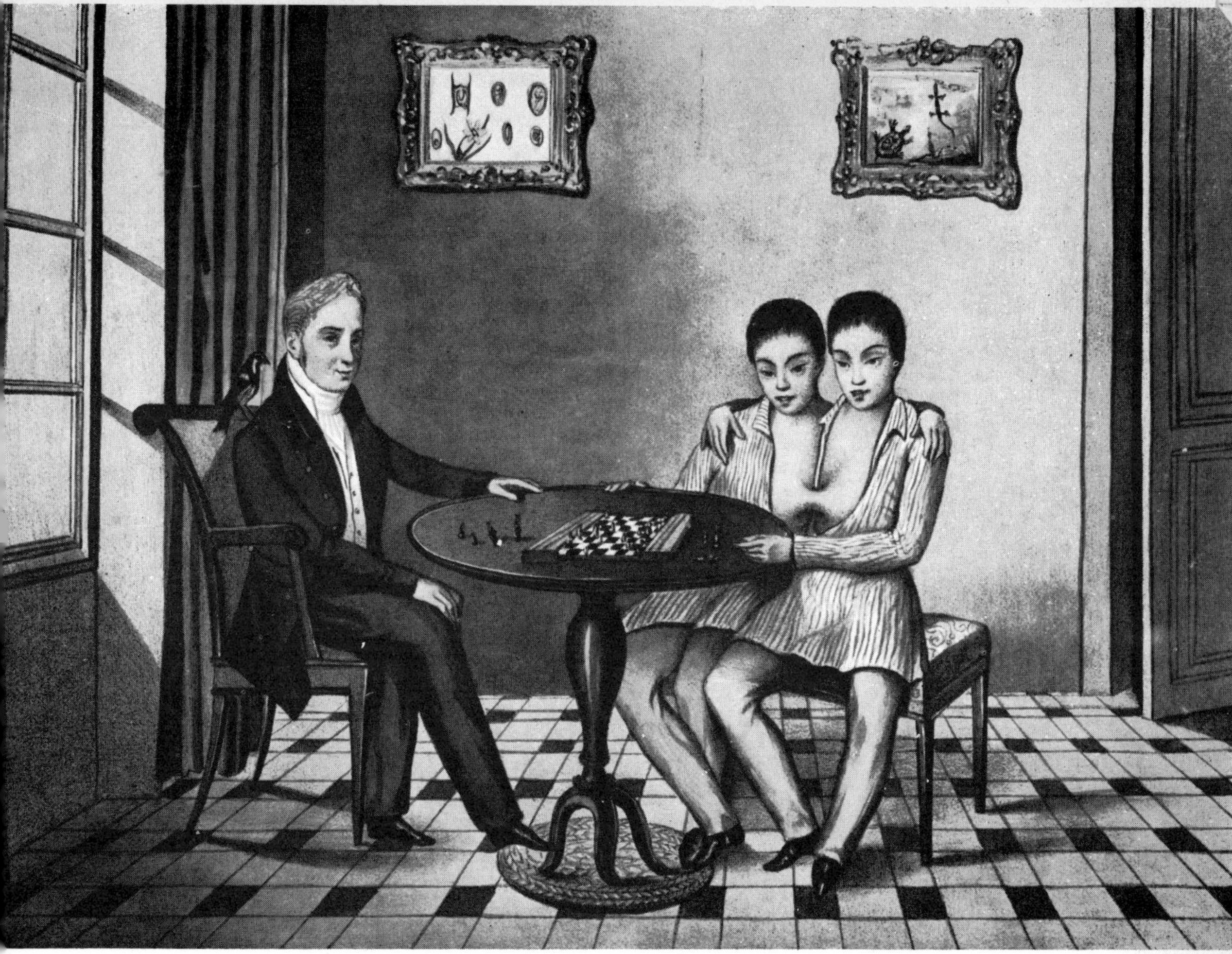

a pathological hatred of each other, so that they had decided to consult the best surgeons in Europe with a view to being surgically separated. But it seems more likely that they thought there was a good prospect of refilling their treasury from further exhibition across the Atlantic. They were, in fact, too old and unfit for a major operation at that time. Chang in particular was drinking too much and was becoming paralysed in one side of his body. They died within three hours of each other on 17 January 1874, and the College of Physicians in Philadelphia sent a commission to perform an autopsy. It was found that their livers were connected through the band which joined them. ¶ A similar band joined Radica and Doddica, known as 'the Orissa Sisters', who were born in India after the sixth pregnancy of their mother in 1889. At the age of four they were

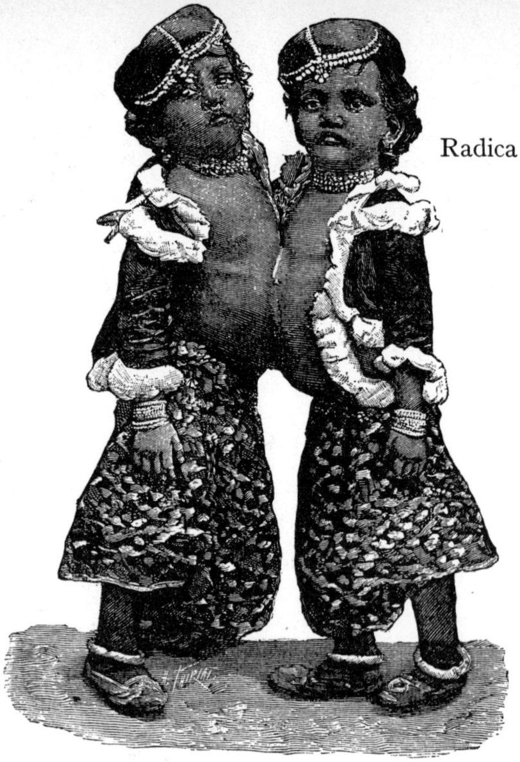

Radica and Doddica, 'the Orissa Sisters', from a contemporary engraving.

brought to Europe, and when they were older they, too, entered show business and went on tour. No operation for the separation of Siamese twins had yet been successful, but a Parisian doctor, Doyen, determined to have another try, and the exercise was carried out in the wildest blaze of publicity – Doyen was known as 'the Barnum of surgery'. A promoter proposed that the operation should be done in the Cirque de Paris as the climax of a charity gala allegedly in aid of the girls. Certainly the operation was the first to take place with each stage being recorded by cameras. Dr Doyen was duly photographed making the first incision on the anaesthetized children, and the sisters died amid the glare of flash-powder. ¶ As in the case of Eng and Chang, the union of Siamese twins through a joining band at the breast-bone usually involves junction of such organs as the liver, and union by osseous junction of the bones of the cranium also generally presupposes common organs, so that successful surgical separation is unlikely in such cases. There is another class of Siamese twins where the individuals are separate and well formed, but the point of fusion is a common part which both individuals must necessarily share. This was

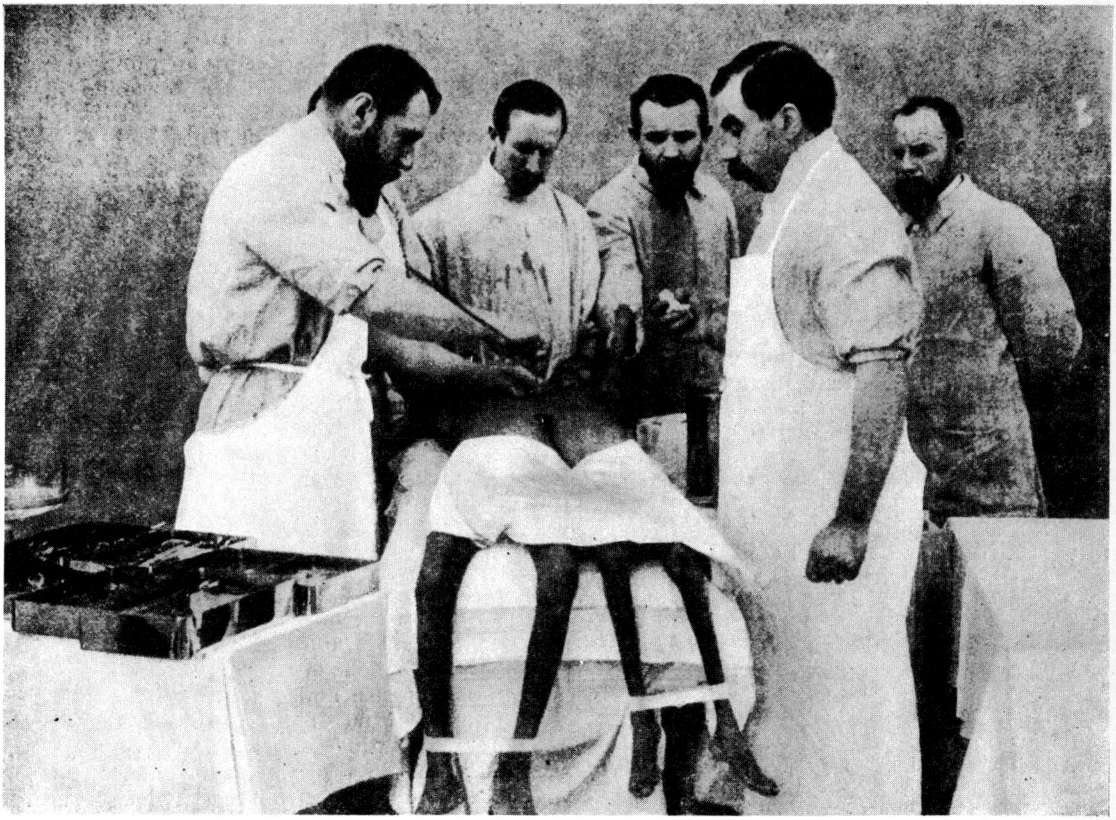

Dr Doyen makes the first incision. . .

the case with the famous 'Biddenden Maids' of Kent, if they ever really existed. One legend concerning them says that they were born at around the time of the accession of Queen Elizabeth I, and that they were joined at the hip and the shoulder, with the central arms being fused into one. This is a most unlikely form of junction, and the details have probably been wrongly transmitted to posterity. Certainly the existence of two sisters in some way physically joined seems a fact, if only from the existence of the Biddenden Maids charity, which each Easter Monday distributed vast quantities of bread and cheese to the poor of the parish, in the name of Eliza and Mary Chalkhurst. And Biddenden cakes were stamped with an old pattern-die showing the two girls apparently joined at shoulder and hip and inscribed with their names and the statement that they had died in the year 1100 at the age of thirty-four. But the die which impressed the legend on the cakes was cut as late as the year 1814, when antiquarian research was not as reliable as it is today, and the Victorian belief that the Biddenden Maids were born in 1066 cannot be substantiated and should not be believed. ¶ It is likely, in spite of the 1814 illustration which follows the legend and shows a junction of the sisters at both the hip and the shoulder, that the Biddenden Maids were in reality separated at the shoulder, with their own arms undeformed, and that they were merely joined at the hip. They would then fall into a recognized classification of terata, the category of pygopagous twins resulting from a junction of the foetuses in the region of the buttocks. In the recorded cases this union has usually been a junction of bone between the sacrum and the coccyx, that is, the area between the place where the backbone joins the pelvis and the tail-bone of the spine itself. ¶ Pygopagous twins recorded have almost always been female and have sometimes shared a common anus and sometimes had separate vaginas but a single vulva. Millie and Christine, born to a Negro slave woman in North Carolina in 1851 and exhibited in the United States and Europe throughout the Victorian era, had separate parts but, though they ate separately, they generally felt hunger and thirst at the same time, and defecated and urinated simultaneously on most occasions. One, sleeping quietly, would be

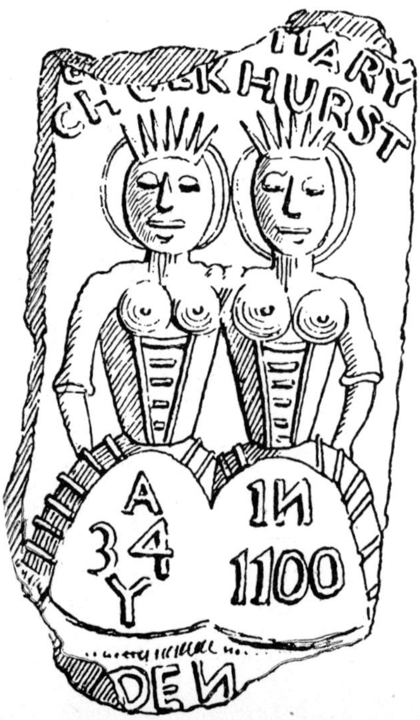

Biddenden Maids' cake,
showing the die cut in 1814.

wakened by a call of nature of the other. Physically, Millie was the weaker – Christine could bend over and lift Millie by the bond of union – but Millie had the stronger will and the dominating spirit. One, from long habit, yielded instinctively to the other's movement, thus preserving the necessary harmony. They had individual thoughts, and carried on distinct conversations at the same time. They were slightly under normal size, were intelligent and physically attractive. They walked, ran, and danced without difficulty and with appreciable grace. On the stage they sang duets with pleasant voices and accompanied themselves with a guitar. ¶ Rosa and Josepha Blazek, 'the Bohemian Twins', whose baby, fathered by the adventurous Viennese butcher, has already been mentioned, were born in 1878. The pictures show them as children and at the height of their theatrical fame. They were joined in the lower part of the lumbar region, and the pelvis was completely fused. They had a common urethral and anal aperture, but a double vaginal orifice, separated by a septum. Sensation was distinct in each, except where the pelvises joined. Rosa, the girl who bore the baby, was the stronger, and when she walked or ran forward she drew her sister after her. Josepha had therefore to proceed backwards. They had independent thoughts and separate minds. One could

The Blazek Sisters as children, and at the height of their theatrical acclaim.

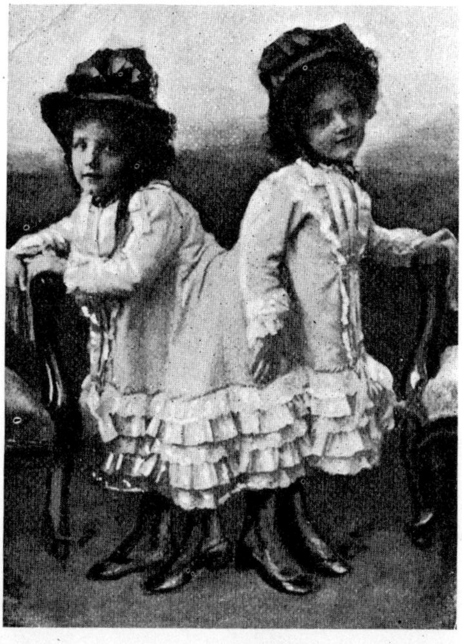

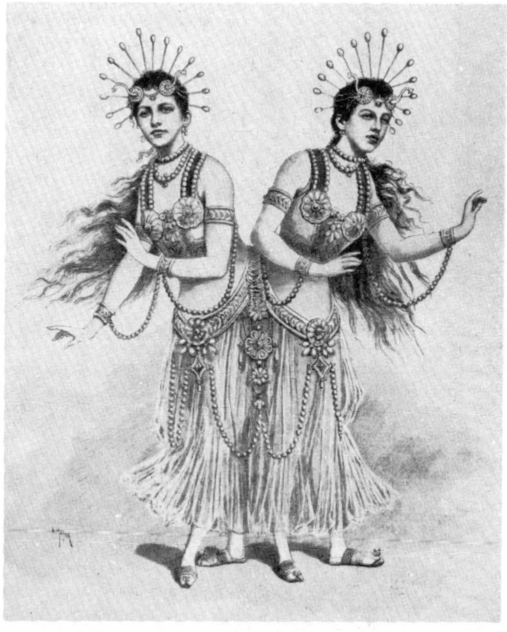

sleep while the other was awake. Many of their tastes were different, one preferring beer and the other wine, one enjoying salad while the other hated it. This was also the case with a similar pair of twin sisters born in 1895. They had two vaginas, two urethras, but a double rectum divided by a septum. They urinated independently but defecated simultaneously. ¶ The Jones twin sisters, born in Indiana in 1889, were described in the contemporary *American Journal of Obstetrics*. They were joined longitudinally by their spinal columns. They had different complexions and their eyes and hair were of different colours. They were publicly exhibited, but they died at the age of twenty months. ¶ The best documentation, from an anatomical point of view, of twins born from the fusion of foetuses below the navel, with common lower parts, exists for two Sardinian sisters, Ritta and Christina, who were joined at the trunk in the region of the waist. The right one, Ritta, was feeble and of a sad disposition, with a melancholy face. Christina was gay and active with a happy face. They suckled at different times, but expelled urine and faeces simultaneously. Their parents quickly earned a small fortune by exhibiting them in Paris, but the exhibition was stopped by the authorities because of the effect it was feared the sight of them might have on pregnant women among the spectators. (This ban was also extended to cover Chang and Eng, the Siamese twins, who were never put on public exhibition in France.) Since the parents of Ritta and Christina were soon reduced to poverty again, and compelled to live in a freezing apartment, Ritta began to fade and it seemed clear that she would not live. At the moment when she died, Christina was suckling at her mother's breast, but she suddenly relaxed and died with a sigh. Doctors had to resort to extraordinary deception to secure a post-mortem, for the authorities had ordered that the bodies should be burned. The eventual dissection showed that the pericardium (the membrane structure surrounding the heart) was single, enclosing two hearts. The digestive organs were double, and separate as far as the lower third of the ilium (the bony hip-girdle). The

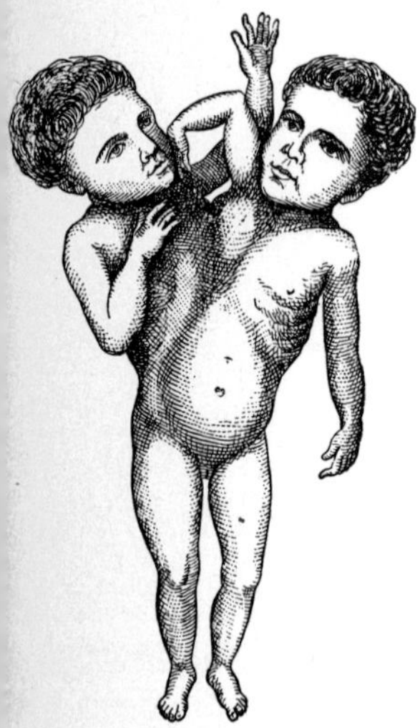

Ritta and Christina, the Sardinian sisters.

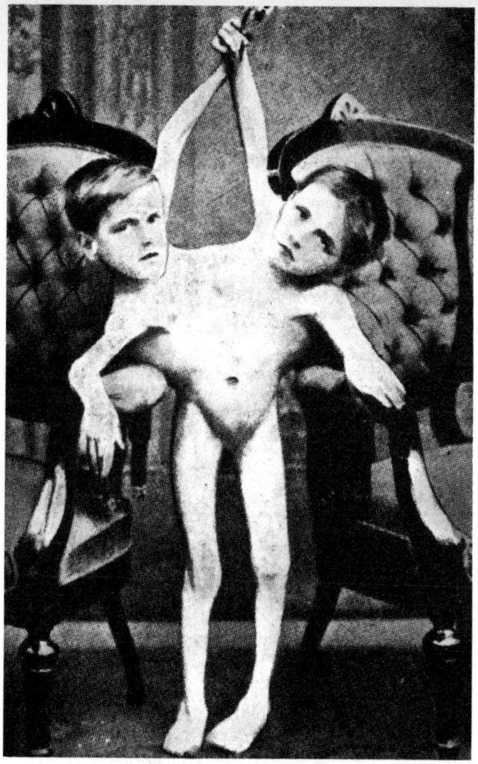

The Tocci brothers: 'every photograph of them shows that they were supporting themselves by a chair'.

livers were fused and the uterus was double. ¶ In the mid-Victorian period the rather similarly disposed Tocci brothers lived on well past infancy and went on the stage to appear, apparently unescorted, in public exhibitions in various parts of Europe. In fact, however, they could not walk, and every photograph of them shows that they were supporting themselves by a chair. They were born near Turin in 1877. Each had a well-formed head, and arms of a normal length but, through obvious lack of exercise, inadequate development, and each had a perfect thorax (chest cavity) as far as the sixth rib. Through merging in the trunk, they had a common abdomen, two legs, a single anus, and one penis, but they had three buttocks, the central one displaying a rudimentary anus. Baptized Giovanni-Battista and Giacomo, they had individual and independent sensations and emotions, but each individual had power only over the leg on his own side and consequently, since they were without co-ordination, they could not walk. ¶ A well-defined category in medical literature is the abnormality termed parasitic terata, which comprises monsters who display a perfect body from which hangs part of a second body, generally issuing from the region of the belly. These have been regularly reported through the centuries by responsible observers. The classic case is undoubtedly that of Lazarus-Joannes Baptista Colloredo, described and illustrated by Bartholinus in his seventeenth-century history of anatomical curiosities. Colloredo was born in Genoa in 1617 and became exceedingly well known through exhibiting himself all over Europe. From his epigastrium, the abdominal wall covering the stomach, there hung an imperfectly developed twin which had one thigh, a trunk with hands and arms, and a well-formed head with a normal growth of hair. The parasite displayed signs of independent existence, such as breathing, but its eyes were closed, and, although saliva dribbled from the open mouth, nothing was ever ingested through it. The genitals were imperfect, and the hands, at the end of comparatively shapely arms, were malformed. Colloredo lived for a

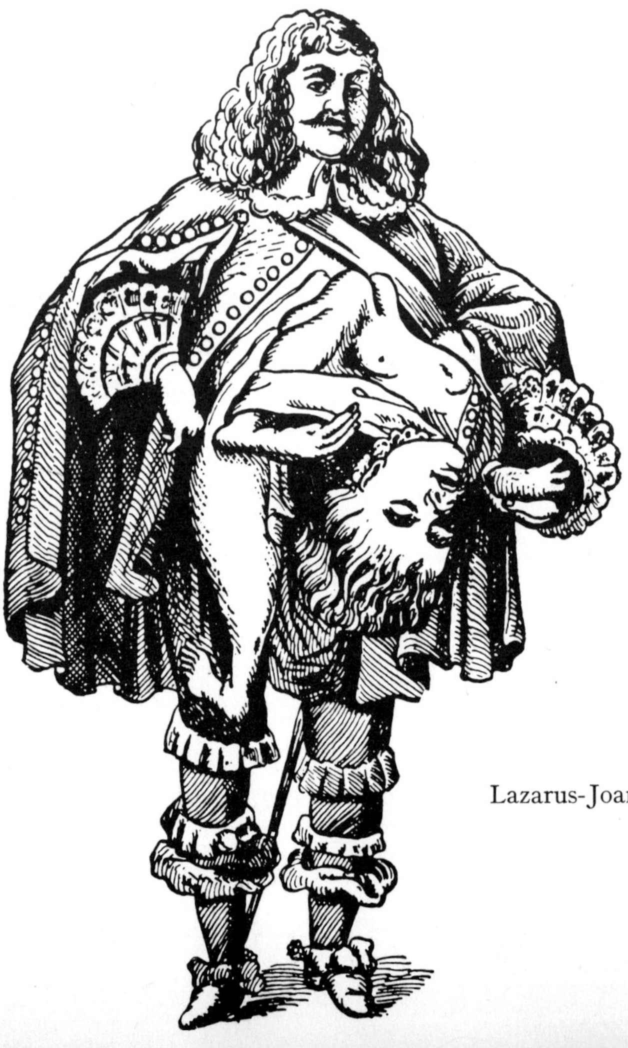

Lazarus-Joannes Baptista Colloredo.

normal span of life, and when he was examined in Scotland at the age of twenty-five was said to be the father of several children, all of whom were normally developed. ¶ Many parasitic terata were reported in Victorian times, including a lady, Madame Louise L., known as 'the woman with four legs', who lived as normal a life as possible in spite of her disability. When she was born in 1869 a second, rudimentary pelvis was attached to her normal pelvis and this carried two atrophied parasitic legs. When Madame Louise had grown to maturity this parasite weighed some 17 lb. Where it joined the main body there were two rudimentary breasts, one larger than the other. No genitalia were seen on it, but the attachment almost obliterated the normal vulva, and the perineum was displaced far backward. Nevertheless, Madame Louise married, and, after two years of apparent infertility, bore two well-formed daughters within a period of three years. ¶ In the 1890s a popular exhibit in the travelling freak-shows was Laloo, then about twenty years old. He had been born in India, but had been shrewdly shipped to the more affluent West. From the lower right side of his breastbone a parasite was attached by a bony stalk, and it was further attached lower down by a more fleshy link apparently containing organs including intestines. The anus of the parasite was not perforated, but there was a well-developed penis, a luxuriant growth of pubic hair, yet no testicles. The penis of the parasite was said to show erection at times, and urine passed through it apparently without Laloo being previously aware of it. In the true spirit of Victorian Grotesque, Laloo's exhibition manager dressed the parasite as a female and said they were showing a brother-and-sister, but there was no trace at all of female characteristics in the parasite. ¶ Abnormal humans showing a duplication of the legs have also been consistently reported throughout medical history. In 1888 the American Professor Wells published a description of the case of Mrs B., together with a photograph, in the *Journal of Obstetrics*. Then comparatively healthy at the age of twenty, Mrs B. was normally shaped above the waist, but the spinal column became divided

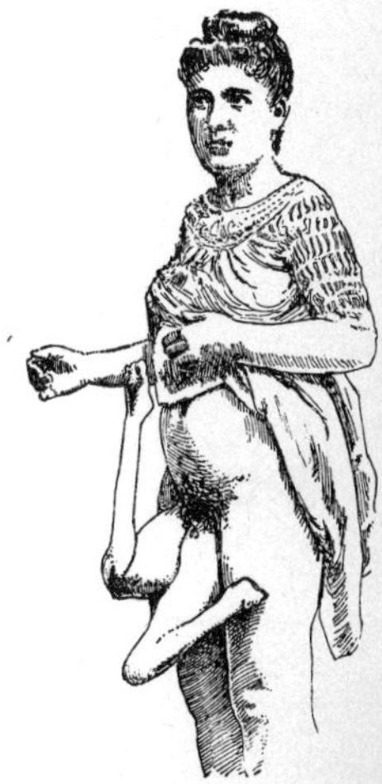

Madame Louise.

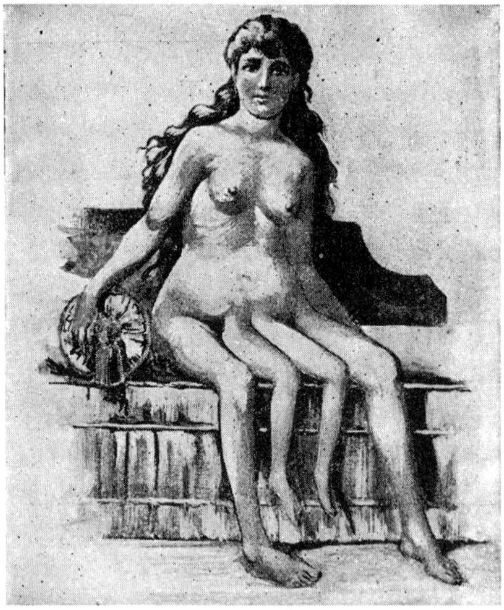

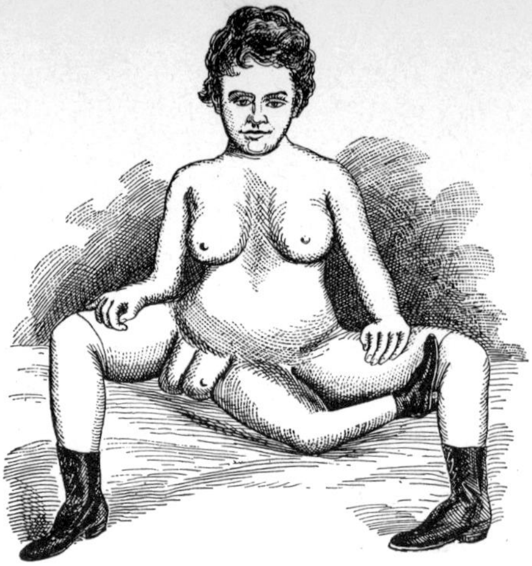

LEFT
Blanche Dumas, born in 1860.

RIGHT
Mrs B, as reported by Professor Wells.

at the third lumbar vertebra, and below this point everything was duplicated. Urination and defecation occurred at different times, but menstruation occurred simultaneously. She had been married at nineteen, and a year later she became pregnant on the left side. But at the fourth month abortion was induced because of the patient's persistent nausea and the expectation of an impossible delivery. Mrs B.'s own doctor, commenting later on this case, said that the lady used her outside legs for walking. He reported that when he had told her that she was pregnant on the left side she had replied, 'I think you are mistaken. If it had been on my right side I would come nearer believing it.' Dr Whaley further questioned his patient and established that her right genitals were almost invariably used for coitus. ¶ Writing in the *British Medical Journal* of January 1889, Dr Bechlinger described a woman of twenty-five, a native of Martinique, who had a third leg attached to a continuation of the tail-bone of the spine and hanging between her legs. The woman had normal breast development above, but where the third leg joined the crutch there were two further rudimentary breasts, each bearing a nipple. There were two vaginas and two well-developed vulvas, both having equally developed sensations. The sexual appetite was markedly strong, and coitus was practised in each vagina. This woman is almost certainly identical with Blanche Dumas, born in 1860, whose case was described elsewhere in Victorian medical literature. ¶ There have been many well-established cases of diphallic terata, that is, the incidence of two penises in a male, and rarely the occurrence of a forked member is described. Over-active imaginations have endowed such males with an exaggerated function, but the specialists have established that virile power diminishes almost invariably in exact proportion to the extent of duplication. Jenisch of Stuttgart illustrated the condition of one diphallic infant. Each penis dribbled urine, draining its separate urethra, and there was a duplication of each scrotum; but only one testicle was observed in each. The most celebrated diphallic in Victorian times was Juan Baptista dos Santos, of Havana, who was born with two over-sized penises and an additional limb between his legs. In 1865 at the age of twenty-two he was said to be possessed of extraordinary animal passion, the mere sight of a female being sufficient to excite him, and to use both penises, after finishing with one continuing with the other. But later observers have cast doubt on this attribution, since it does not agree with other, later descriptions of dos Santos, in which no excessive sexual ability was mentioned. Apart from this proclivity, the man's mental and physical functions were

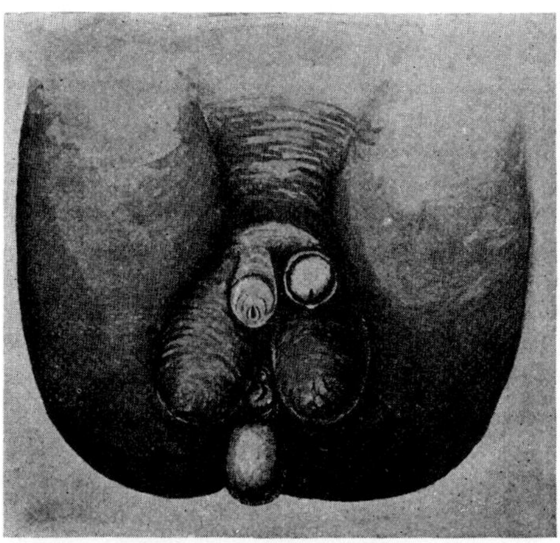

Jenisch's case of a diphallic infant.

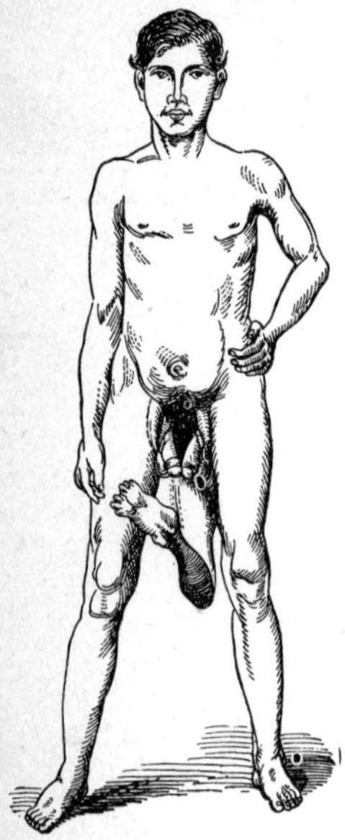

developed above normal, and he impressed everybody with his accomplishments. ¶ Duplication of the penis as the only abnormality in a male is very seldom recorded, only some twenty cases being described in teratologic literature. It is far more generally allied with other major deformities and duplications, most commonly encountered with an atresia (lack of normal passage) in the anus. A well-nigh incredible but nevertheless solidly authenticated abnormality is *foetus in foetu*, the bizarre occurrence of an infant carrying within its own body the foetus of a twin, and finally delivering it at a much later date. It has been likened to the eventuality of a man being pregnant with his own brother or sister, and certainly the occurrence of *foetus in foetu* is as likely in the male body as the female. In one sense it is the accomplishment of the old myth according to which Eve was born from Adam:

Juan Baptista dos Santos.

> And the Lord God caused a deep sleep to fall upon Adam, and he slept: and he took one of his ribs, and closed up the flesh instead thereof; and the rib, which the Lord God had taken from man, made he a woman, and brought her unto the man. And Adam said, This is now bone of my bones, and flesh of my flesh: she shall be called Woman, because she was taken out of Man. Therefore shall a man leave his father and his mother, and shall cleave unto his wife: and they shall be one flesh.

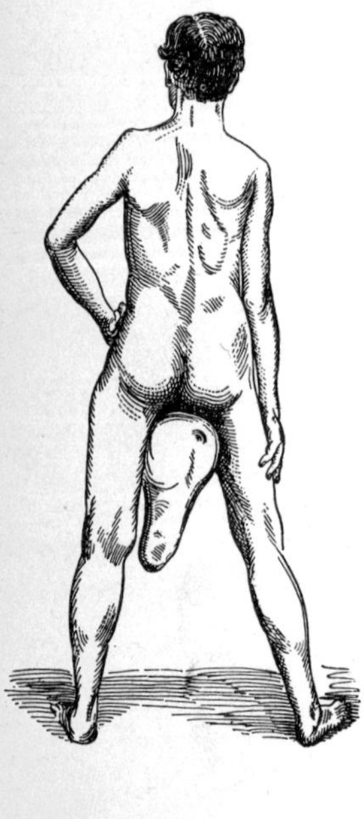

Many ancient writers spoke of the occurrence of *foetus in foetu*. In 1723, when the documentation of science had acquired more credibility, Ruysch described a tumour contained in the body of a man which was composed of hair, molar teeth, and other evidence of a foetus. In 1748 Huxham reported to the Royal Society the history of a child which, when born, had a tumour near the anus larger than its whole body, and this tumour contained rudiments of an embryo. Gaetano-Nocito, quoted in the nineteenth-century *Dictionnaire des sciences médicales*, gave the history of a man of twenty-seven who was seized with great pain in the right hypochondrium (the stomach wall below the ribs) and from this place there issued subsequently foetal bones and a mass of macerated embryo. His mother had had several double pregnancies, and from the length of the respective tibiae

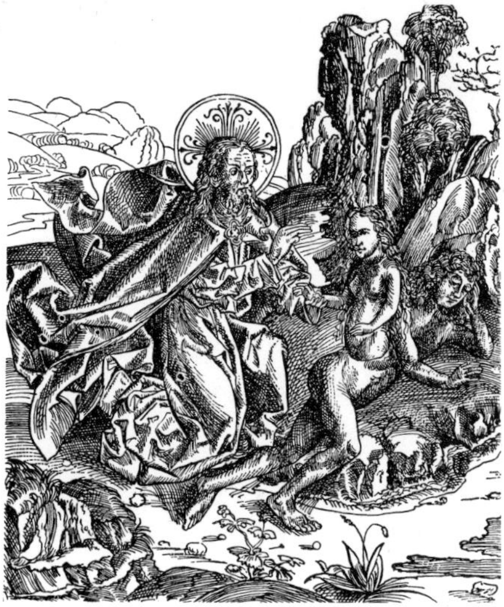

The Birth of Eve from an old engraving.

(shin-bones) one of the foetuses seemed to be of two months' and the other of three months' intra-uterine life. The man died five years after the abscess had burst spontaneously. ¶ Blundell reported in the *Lancet* that he had known 'a boy who was literally and without evasion with child, for the foetus was contained in a sac communicating with the abdomen and was connected to the side of the cyst by a short umbilical cord; nor did the foetus make its appearance until the boy was eight or ten years old, when after much enlargement of pregnancy and subsequent flooding the boy died'. The foetus was removed after death and was found to be not very imperfectly formed, having the size of about six or seven months' gestation. In 1891 several popular newspapers took up a story originating in Mexico City regarding a 'Man-Mother' from whose body a skilful surgeon had extracted a 'perfectly developed foetus'. In the absence of photographic illustration to a topical story of this nature, a wood-cut was syndicated showing a tumour on a man's back which had been opened revealing a crying baby. Two years later the *Universal Medical Journal* of Philadelphia printed an article by a specialist in teratology named Rodriguez which explained the true facts of this exaggerated story. An Indian boy aged twenty-two presented a tumour in the sacrococcygeal region measuring 53 centimetres in circumference at the base, having a vertical diameter of 17 centimetres and a transverse diameter of 13 centimetres. This tumour had been present since birth, at which time it was about the size of a pigeon's egg. Rodriguez, who had been studying terata of this kind in Mexico, diagnosed a dermoid cyst and conducted two surgical operations on the boy, who died after the second. The contents of the cyst verified the diagnosis. A dermoid cyst is not a recognizable foetus but is a mass of skin, hair, bones, and even teeth among sebaceous matter. ¶ Hermaphrodites are double-sexed creatures. Their existence has been reported since antiquity, and they are now recognized as presenting a major teratum. Most reported cases are not true hermaphrodites, but persons with a malformation of the external genitalia. A prolonged clitoris, prolapsed (fallen) ovaries, masculine configuration, and excessive hairiness have accounted for many supposed cases of hermaphroditism in females, while in males, a cleft scrotum, an ill-developed penis, hypospadias or epispadias (conditions in which the urethra opens into the front or back of the shaft of the penis), development of breasts, or feminization of the contour of the body have prompted false reports of 'double sex'. Some cases have, however, been proved by dissection to have been true hermaphrodites, when the entire genitalia of both sexes have been found in one body. ¶ Catherine/Charles Hoffman changed sex in 1870 at the age of forty-six. She had previously been considered a female. She had menstruated late, at the age of nineteen, but her breasts were well formed and she had the sexual instincts of a woman, and lived with a male lover for twenty years. Then her sexual desires changed, and she attempted coitus with a woman, with such evident satisfaction that she married a woman soon afterwards. Fitch reported in the *New York Medical Journal* of 20 November 1890 the case of a twenty-eight-year-old house-servant of masculine appearance who was arrested by the police for violating the laws of prostitution. On examination, well-developed male and female genital organs were found. The labia majora were normal, the vagina was spacious and discharged mucus in a profuse leucorrhea. She stated that several years previously she had given birth to a normal child. In place of a clitoris she had a penis which, in erection, measured $5\frac{1}{4}$ inches long and $3\frac{5}{8}$ inches in circumference. The glans penis and the urethra were perfectly formed. The scrotum contained two testicles, each about an inch long. The mons veneris was sparsely covered with straight black hair. She claimed functional ability with both sets of genitals and said she experienced equal sexual gratification with either. Semen issued from the penis, and every three weeks she had a short menstruation. ¶ In the autumn of 1864 a sick patient came to the Hôtel-Dieu, the traditional old public hospital in Paris, clearly needing treatment for chronic pleurisy. In many aspects, including baldness, the patient gave the appearance of a long-bearded old man. He said he was sixty-five years old and had long scraped a miserable living as a mountebank. He added that in early life he had been taken for a woman. He had menstruated at eight years old, and had been examined by a panel of doctors in puberty. This patient was Marie-Madeleine Lefort, on whom a full report had been made to the Paris Faculté de Médicine in the year of Waterloo. She was then said to be nineteen years of age. She had well-developed breasts with erectile nipples surrounded by a brown areola from which

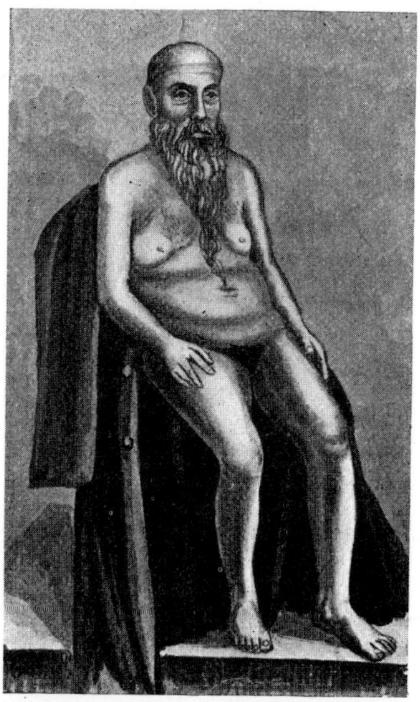

Marie-Madeleine Lefort,
at sixty-five years of age.

issued several hairs. Her pelvis was large and her thighs were shaped like those of a woman. Projecting from the vulva was a body looking like a penis, 7 centimetres long and slightly erectile at times. It had a mobile foreskin but it was not perforated. She had a vulva with two well-shaped labia and there was an opening at the root of the clitoris. She menstruated slightly. However, the area of the face below the ears showed some sign of sprouting the beginnings of a beard, and she wore a shaped dark moustache on her upper lip. This was the curious but glowing young body which became, almost fifty years later, the pathetically sick shell of humanity at the Hôtel-Dieu. Lefort died at the hospital within two months, and an autopsy on that bald and bearded body showed that all the essentials of female sexuality – uterus, ovaries, Fallopian tubes – though with an abnormality in the process of the urethra, were present in the earthly remains of the departed mountebank. ¶ By strict definition true hermaphroditism cannot be declared until the doctors have failed to declare a sex – that is, they cannot maintain, where two sets of genitals are discovered, that the function of one sex predominates over the other. Much more common than true hermaphoditism is so-called spurious hermaphroditism, and in the majority of instances the initial doubt has been caused by elongation of the clitoris – in one extreme case recorded in 1851, the year of the Great Exhibition, to a length of 5 inches and a thickness of 1 inch. Spurious hermaphroditism does not imply any intention to deceive on the part of the sufferer from this condition, and it is a label with unpleasant moral overtones, since the unfortunate fact is that often only the death and dissection of the subject will enable the last word to be said on whether the deceased was a true or a spurious hermaphrodite. ¶ Hermaphroditism was shown to be a hereditary condition in some circumstances. In 1885 Pozzi recorded in the *Gazette médicale de Paris* a family of nine individuals in whom spurious hermaphroditism was observed. The first in the family was a female who had had four children. The second had been christened a female but was probably a male. The third, fourth, and fifth had been born apparently normal but had died young. The sixth was a female with St Vitus' dance who was, in addition, feeble-minded and, at the age of twenty-nine, had one illegitimate child. The seventh was a healthy male who had married. The eighth had been christened a female, but after a history of difficult acceptance had been examined by the Faculty of Medicine and had been declared to be a male. The ninth had been christened a female, but on examination at the age of eighteen was found to have male genitals, though the breasts were well developed. ¶ Such a confused brotherhood/sisterhood would doubtless qualify without question for the title 'problem family'. Eugenic fears that the race would be degenerated by reproduction from stock of this quality may, however, be largely discounted. Although popular mythology credits hermaphrodites not only with dual facility but with doubled lust (and the case of the 'ambidextrous' servant from New York may seem to bear this out), the best authorities on the subject contend that in almost all cases hermaphrodites are sterile. In addition many of them have been declared sexually indifferent, and long observation by the specialists has tended to show that the sexual appetite diminishes in proportion to the imperfections in the genitalia. In Victorian times the teratologists established what they believed to be a law of evolution in hermaphroditism which prevented perfection: if one section of the genitals was extraordinarily developed, the other part would be correspondingly atrophied. Thus, in the case of extreme development of the clitoris they would expect to find an imperfectly developed uterus or ovaries. And this, they said, would be one of the causes of the sterility met in these cases.

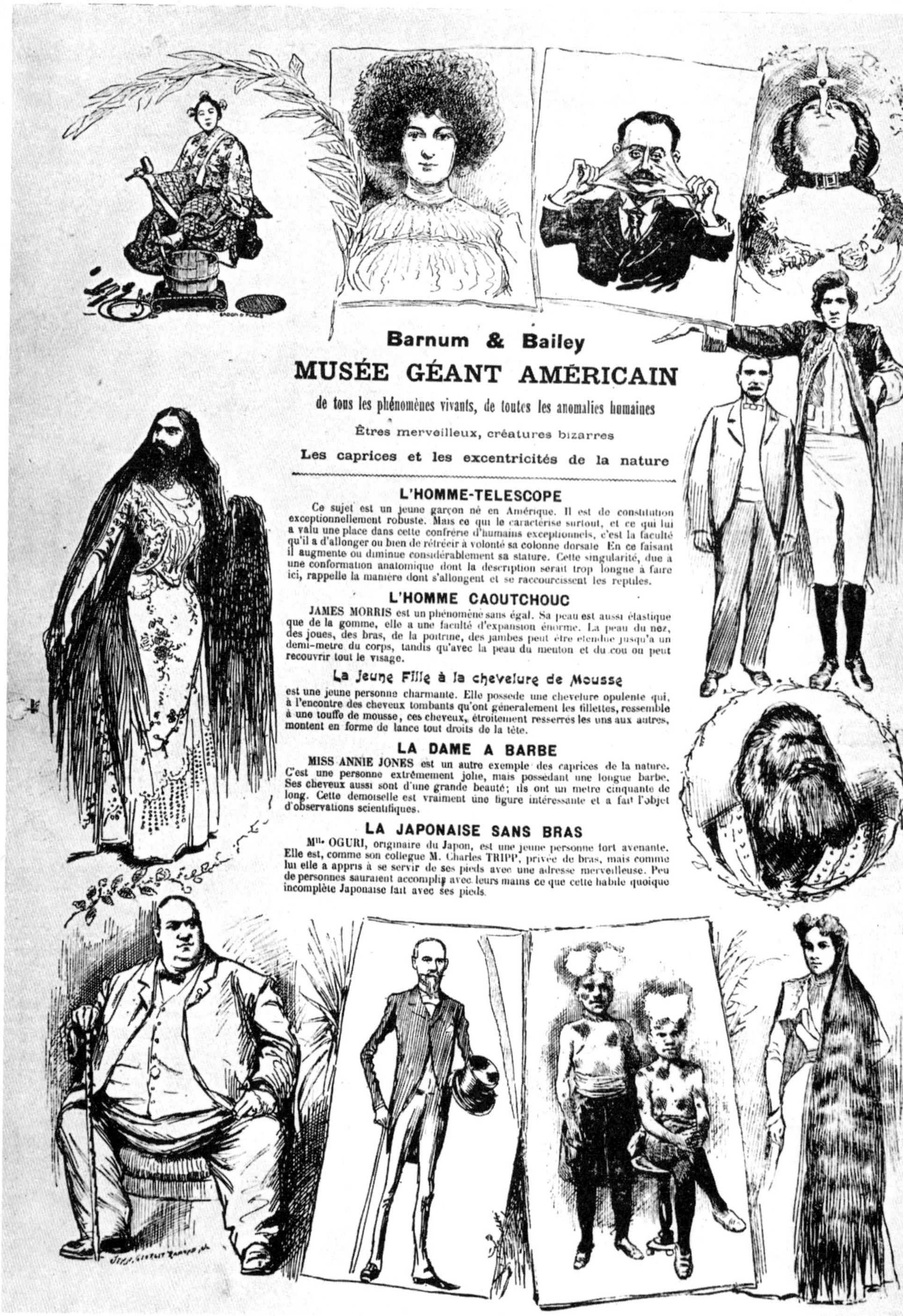
Barnum & Bailey
MUSÉE GÉANT AMÉRICAIN
de tous les phénomènes vivants, de toutes les anomalies humaines
Êtres merveilleux, créatures bizarres
Les caprices et les excentricités de la nature
L'HOMME-TELESCOPE
Ce sujet est un jeune garçon né en Amérique. Il est de constitution exceptionnellement robuste. Mais ce qui le caractérise surtout, et ce qui lui a valu une place dans cette confrérie d'humains exceptionnels, c'est la faculté qu'il a d'allonger ou bien de rétrécir à volonté sa colonne dorsale En ce faisant il augmente ou diminue considérablement sa stature. Cette singularité, due à une conformation anatomique dont la description serait trop longue à faire ici, rappelle la manière dont s'allongent et se raccourcissent les reptiles.
L'HOMME CAOUTCHOUC
JAMES MORRIS est un phénoméne sans égal. Sa peau est aussi élastique que de la gomme, elle a une faculté d'expansion énorme. La peau du nez, des joues, des bras, de la poitrine, des jambes peut être etendue jusqu'a un demi-metre du corps, tandis qu'avec la peau du menton et du cou on peut recouvrir tout le visage.
La Jeune Fille à la chevelure de Mousse
est une jeune personne charmante. Elle possede une chevelure opulente qui, à l'encontre des cheveux tombants qu'ont géneralement les fillettes, ressemble à une touffe de mousse, ces cheveux, étroitement resserrés les uns aux autres, montent en forme de lance tout droits de la tête.
LA DAME A BARBE
MISS ANNIE JONES est un autre exemple des caprices de la nature. C'est une personne extrêmement jolie, mais possédant une longue barbe. Ses cheveux aussi sont d'une grande beauté; ils ont un metre cinquante de long. Cette demoiselle est vraiment une figure intéressante et a fait l'objet d'observations scientifiques.
LA JAPONAISE SANS BRAS
Mlle. OGURI, originaire du Japon, est une jeune personne fort avenante. Elle est, comme son collegue M. Charles TRIPP, privée de bras, mais comme lui elle a appris à se servir de ses pieds avec une adresse merveilleuse. Peu de personnes sauraient accomplir avec leurs mains ce que cette habile quoique incomplète Japonaise fait avec ses pieds.

A French advertising bill for a Barnum and Bailey tour.

CHAPTER THREE

DESPERATE BUT NOT SERIOUS

THERE HAVE AWAYS BEEN two ways in which to react to adversity. These were best illustrated in Victorian times by the contrasting reactions of the inhabitants of two capitals to the crises, wars, revolutions, annexations, and assassinations of the troubled nineteenth century. The Berliners were handled with somewhat heavy duplicity by means of bureaucratic bulletins clumsily designed to prevent the population from panicking; the tenor of these communiqués was always 'The situation is serious, but not desperate.' The gayer Viennese used to make up their own communiqués, and the pronouncements were always the same: 'The situation is desperate, but not serious.' That is probably the best way to accept those blemishes and abnormalities which, because they are not necessarily fatal to a new-born child, are classified by the experts as *minor terata* (though to sensitive sufferers the affliction can be excessively serious). Blessed were they with the temperament to recognize that, if surgical action or drug therapy was out of the question, what could start as a diverting but not too rewarding parlour trick might be put to more lucrative use in a circus – that, at any rate, was the attitude in Victorian times. Today exhibitors as well as spectators are far more sensitive. Yet the fact still remains that these terata *are* wonders, and ordinary people as well as medical specialists are behaving only naturally if they develop a profound interest in them. ¶ The 'India-Rubber Man' illustrated on the Barnum & Bailey poster was James Morris and he was declared to be a matchless marvel. His skin was so elastic all over that the nose, the chin, the skin of the arms and legs could be pulled out until it had stretched 18 inches from the body. When the skin was released it sprang back into the original conformation. He could pull out the skin of his chin and neck until it covered the whole of his face. The reason for such cases of abnormal elasticity of the skin is that the skin is fixed extremely loosely to the underlying tissues, and at the same time its elasticity is so great that it can be stretched like rubber. Felix Wehrle, the 'Elastic-Skin Man' illustrated, not only had the power to stretch his skin but could also bend his fingers backwards and forwards. ¶ In congenital cases of this nature there is loose attachment of the skin without

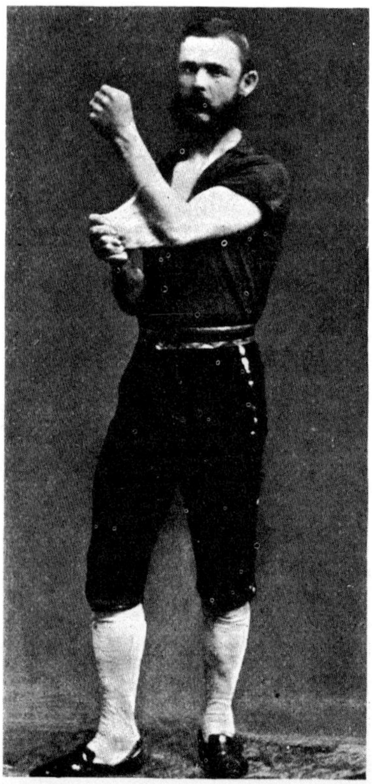

Felix Wehrle, the 'Elastic-Skin Man'.

hypertrophy, or excessive increase in area. The skin is truly elastic in that, when released, it does not return in folds but covers the original site tightly like normal skin. A Dr Seiffert, who had the chance to dissect a subject who had had this attribute, found that beneath the skin the elastic fibres were quite normal, but there was a transformation of the connective tissues of the dermis (the tissue which supports the skin and its appendages such as hair follicles and sweat glands) into an unformed tissue resembling a myxoma (a non-malignant tumour of the connective tissue, containing a sort of mucus). The ordinary bundles of connective tissue were completely absent. Stretching of the skin is, of course, common in cases of obesity and on the bodies of women who have borne many children, notably in the breasts and the abdominal walls. But in these cases the skin consistently falls in folds, and it does not have the normal appearance of the true 'elastic skin' phenomenon. ¶ Occasionally an abnormal development of the scalp can be encountered in which the top of the head is pierced by deep longitudinal furrows. In almost all the cases known to the Victorians the subjects had a congenital brain disability. By the definitions of the time they were idiots. The folds are due to excessive growth in the scalp and the underlying muscles. The same sort of furrowing is noticeable in the scalp of a dog when it pricks its ears, and contemporary thought advanced the theory that this condition was an example of an evolutionary reversion to inferior types. In one case of a man with this abnormal development muscles could be stimulated over which the man had no apparent control. By tickling the scalp over the back of the neck two cross-furrows involuntarily deepened. ¶ The impervious skin of the Indian fakir has long been a cartoon joke. The condition undoubtedly exists, and it has always excited great argument as to whether it is due to a congenital hardness of the skin or to a self-hypnosis which, after long practice, renders the skin insensitive – or to a combination of both. But if the fakir lying on his bed of nails is merely *telling himself* that it does not hurt, why does he not at least bleed? The Victorians used to flock to the London Alhambra music hall when a performer named Rhannin (a native of Ceylon) was billed to appear. He climbed barefoot up a ladder whose rungs were sharp-edged swords. He lay on a bed of nails with four men sitting on him. He curled himself up in a barrel, through the shell of which sharp nails were driven, and he was rolled about the stage at a fast rate inside this barrel. He was a very handsome bronze-skinned man who billed himself as 'The Man with the Iron Skin', and he claimed – for the purposes of show business publicity, at any rate – that he had found an elixir that rendered the human skin impervious to any metal point or sharpened edge of a knife or a dagger. (He did not, however, back up this claim by selling the elixir to shipyard riveters, or to the War Office for issue to infantry battalions before a cavalry charge – which would have been a very profitable venture if the lotion was as practical as he claimed.) His greatest feat, performed in Berlin, was to pass his entire body through a hoop, the inside of which was hardly big enough to admit his body and was closely set with sharp knife-points, daggers, and nails. After this performance the medical profession clamoured to examine him. They were divided as to his immunity, and some declared that he was a fakir who had, through long practice alone, hardened himself against the effect of sharp metal on his skin. But the professors of the Berlin Clinic in a symposium of lectures about the physical condition of Rhannin, declared that the resistance of his skin was inexplicable. ¶ Many performers have claimed immunity from burns and have mounted very impressive acts depending on the handling of fire. But the experts gave them no credit for any abnormal condition of the skin, maintaining that these men were very accomplished fire-jugglers who were exploiting acquired skill rather than a congenital abnormality. ¶ Albinos suffer from an absence of the pigment melanin, which gives a characteristic colour to the skin and the hair. Albinism is now known to be due to a recessive gene in one of the chromosomes. The Victorians who researched it found many instances of heredity influencing albinism, and some believed that it could be the consequence of adverse living

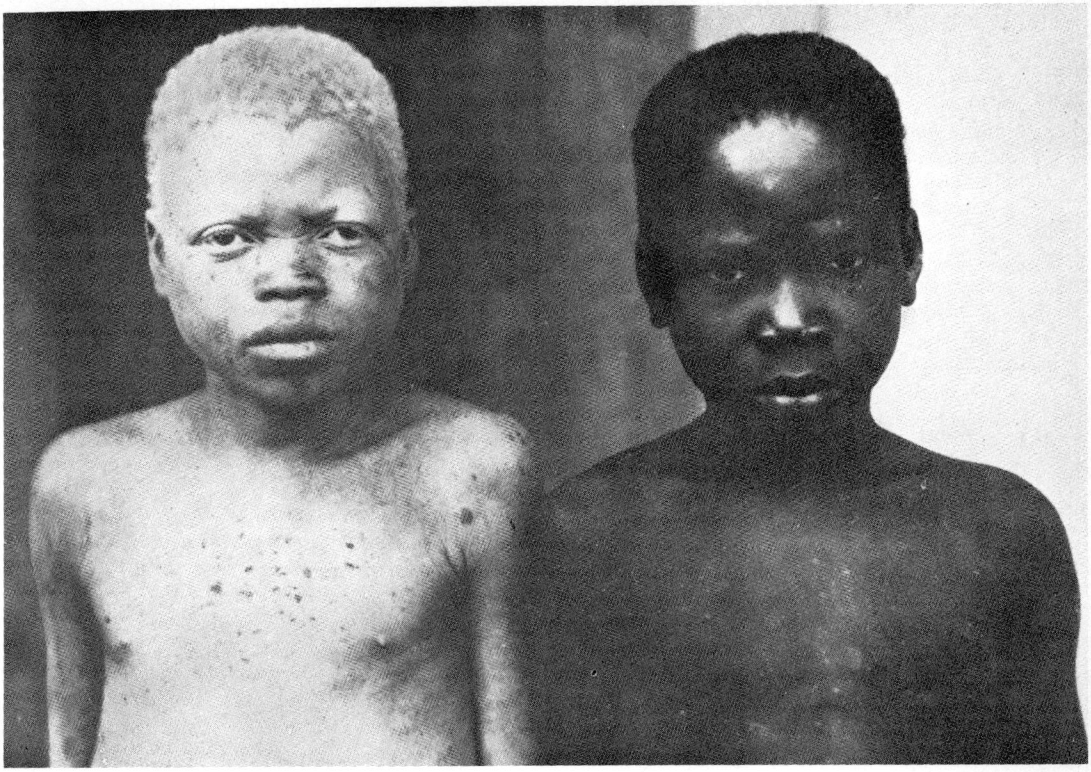

An albino with his brother, from the West Coast of Africa.

conditions caused by poverty, hunger, lack of exercise, and lack of light. Albinism occurs in all races, but it is clearly most remarkable in a Negro. Wherever it occurs the subject has virtually no colouring at all in the skin and hair. The eyebrows and eyelashes are of a brilliant white, or may be yellowish. The iris and the choroid – the (normally) coloured circle surrounding the pupil of the eye, and the middle coat of the eye containing blood-vessels and, normally, pigment – are deprived of colouring matter, and in looking at the eye one sees a rosy zone and a pink pupil. Because their eyes are not protected by pigment, albinos tend to keep their eyes three-quarters closed. Light literally hurts them, and they tend to destroy the refractive power of the retina by crushing the eyeball in their constant endeavour to shut out the light; consequently they suffer from exhaustion of the retina and an involuntary oscillation of the eyeball. When partial albinism occurs the parts most afflected are the genitals, the hair,

George Alexander, a young Negro from the Caribbean. An engraving published in 1809.

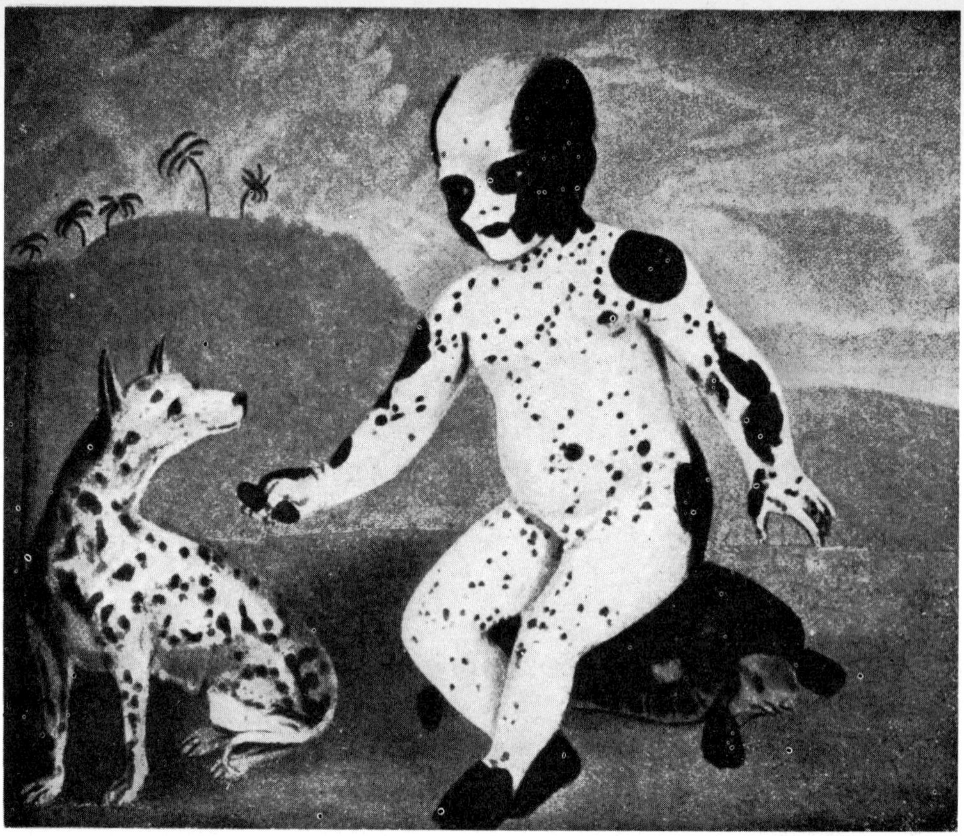

the face, the top of the trunk, the nipples, and the backs of the hands and fingers. Partially albinic Negroes – or 'pied blacks' – became the most common exhibits of this type in travelling shows. Logically, a black and white body could just as well be produced from a localized excess of colouring in a Caucasian, when the anomaly would be the black spots. Partial melanism (the opposite of albinism) due to excessive pigmentation in the tissues and the skin does in fact exist. Total melanism, the complete abnormal darkening of the skin, is unknown in man, however, so that the affliction shows itself only in localized blotching of a different depth of colour. ¶ Human horns are abnormal outgrowths from the skin, and are far more common than is normally supposed. Horns up to 11 inches long and 2½ inches in circumference, taken from human heads, were displayed in nineteenth-century medical museums. The growth of horns – which has always symbolized, not the influence of the Devil, as might be supposed, but the fact that the wearer has an unfaithful

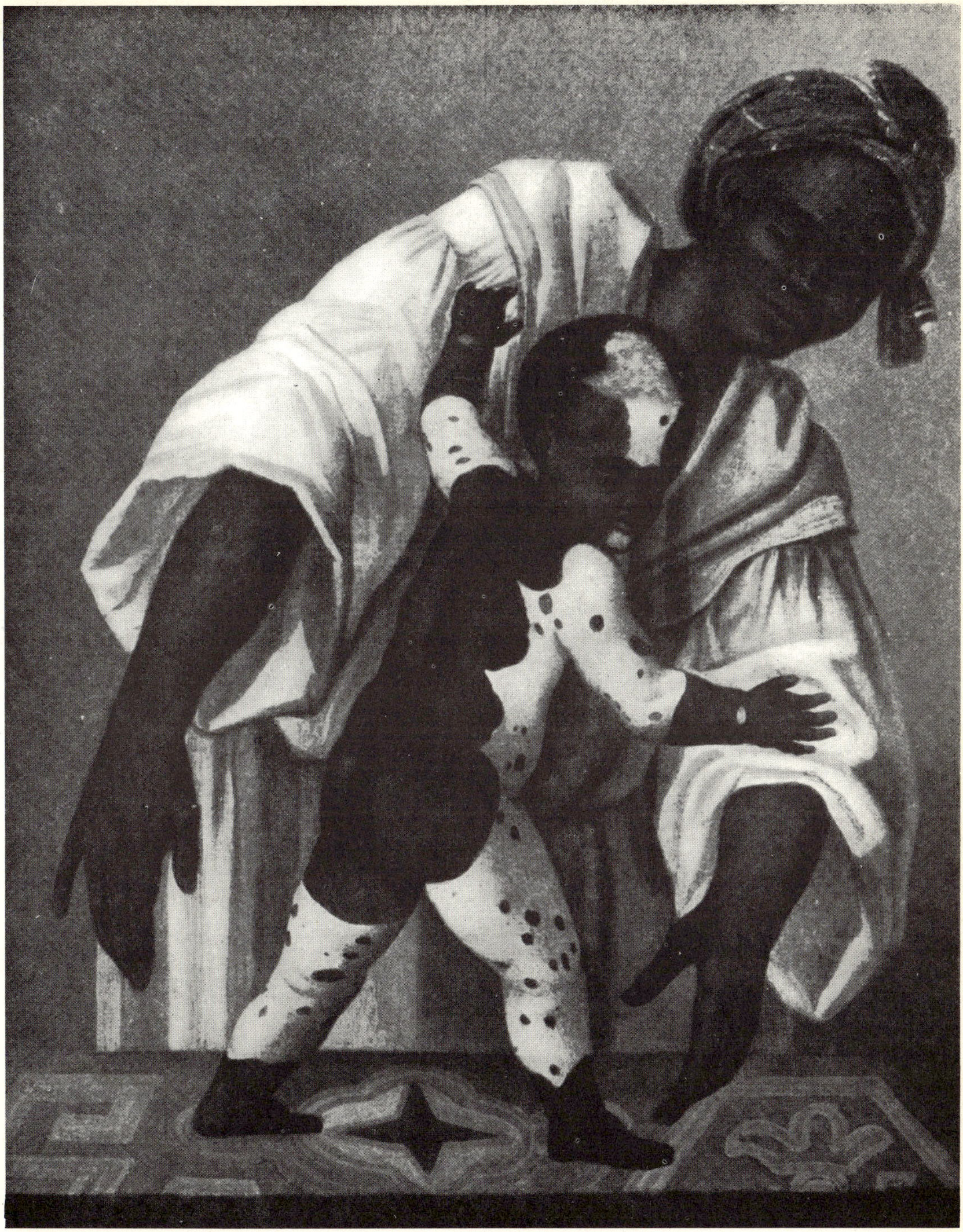

A young albino from Martinique, 1782.

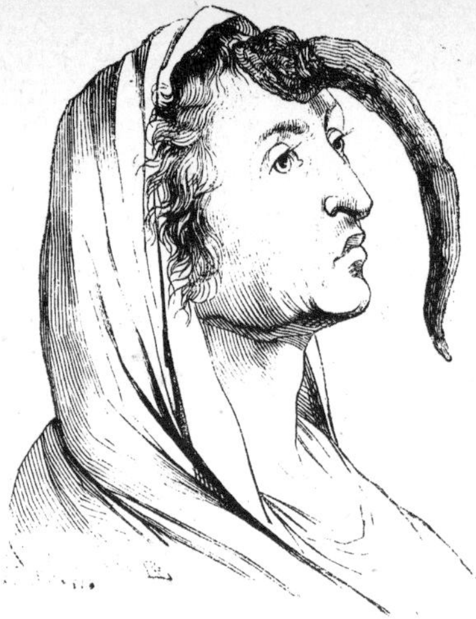

LEFT

The Widow Dimanche of Paris, who became known as 'Mother Horn'.

BELOW

François Trouillu, 'l'homme à la corne'.

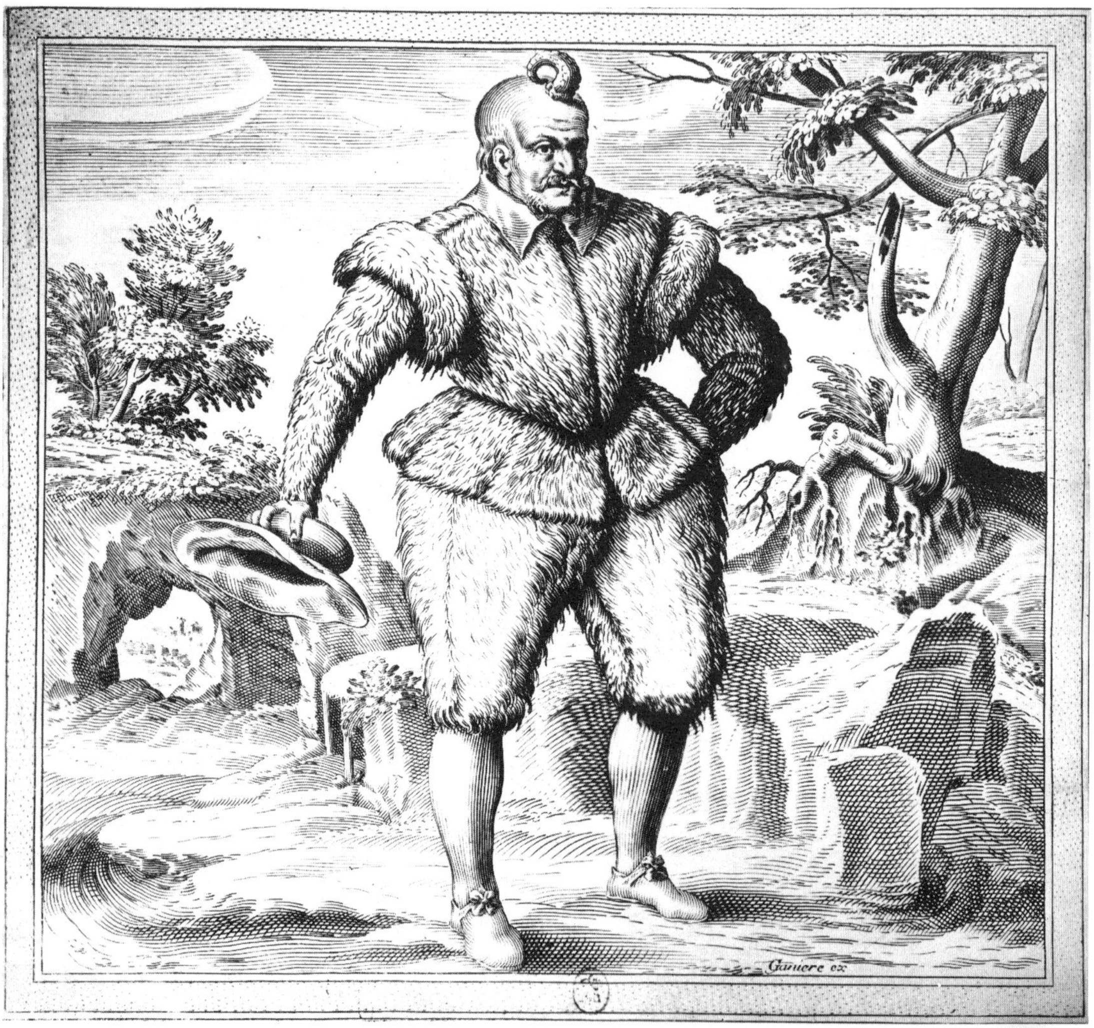

spouse who is cuckolding him or her at the moment – has naturally been a source of the most ribald merriment to all beholders and has been lovingly illustrated from living specimens down through the ages. The upper picture in the accompanying set is of a woman, the Widow Dimanche of Paris, who became known as Mother Horn. (Horns do, in fact, occur on women far more frequently than on men.) Out of 90 instances collected by the Victorian researcher Wilson and reported in the *Medico-Chirurgical Transactions* of London, 48 were on the head, 4 on the face, 4 on the nose, 11 on the thigh, 3 on the leg or foot, 6 on the back, 5 on the penis, and 9 on the trunk. ¶ In 1887 Lamprey reported in the *British Medical Journal* the result of his careful investigations into the then famous phenomenon of the 'Horned Men of Africa'. He found that these horns were caused by a congenital malformation and remarkable development of the infra-orbital ridge of the maxillary bone, the upper jaw-bone. Working through an interpreter he found that the condition was congenital and not the result of any injury or self-inflicted wound, as was then thought to be the case. The protuberances caused little inconvenience and had no disturbing effect on the sense of smell. Lamprey was able to prove that there was no substantiation for the belief that the tribes in West Africa used artificial means to produce this deformity, although it was known that many aboriginal peoples in other parts of the world did so. ¶ Horns have been known to grow in large numbers on the same body, and the record seems to have been held by a woman who had 185 horns. In 1878 Dr Pancoast of Philadelphia wrote about a sea captain whose nose, cheeks, forehead, and lips had been covered with horny growths, most of which had fallen off before he consulted the doctor. The captain was seventy-eight years old and had naturally been exposed to wind and weather all his life. He had suffered three attacks of erysipelas due to prolonged exposure. ¶ Complete baldness is regarded by some of those who display it as a positive sexual attraction. There is little evidence that this was a popular belief in the nineteenth century, which may be categorized as a very hairy age. Complete hairlessness

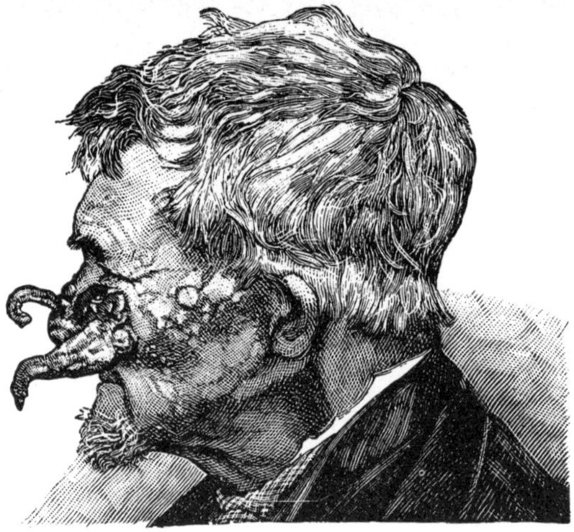

Cutaneous horns and growths in the case related by Dr Pancoast of Philadelphia.

did have its place though as a sexual fetish, but more often in perverse circumstances: the rather exaggeratedly gross form of the hairless eunuch in the Turkish harem became the prototype. And the Victorians were perhaps better aware than has been supposed of the consequences of castration – which may catastrophically curtail the performance but not extinguish the desire, nor diminish the capacity of the body for those rites of sodomy for which the Turks had a deserved reputation. The Turks were also known in Victorian times for their frequent distaste for hair during their more esoteric moments, and they practised depilatory customs, not by shaving, but by the use of ointments and pomades, principally about the genitals. ¶ The male attitude to hairlessness in women has been very variable. The American habit, long since adopted in Great Britain, of masculine approval for women with hairless armpits is even now not fully copied in Mediterranean countries. Many Italian women are still forbidden by their menfolk to shave under the arms, since the hair in its natural state heightens the desire of these particular males. Hair around the genitals has always been the subject of certain sexual cults, and there were well-known Parisian brothels in Victorian times where the pubic hair of the prostitutes was removed – but only in order that the girls could more comfortably wear 'false pussies' of a most luxuriant growth and in more stimulating colours. Rows of these miniature wigs were sometimes to be seen pegged on a clothes line to dry after the day's laundry operations. ¶ Complete hairlessness from birth (known as congenital alopecia) has been a comparatively rarely observed occurrence. Sometimes it is associated with complete lack of teeth. Other instances were recorded by Victorian writers where the condition was allied with an inability either to sweat or to shed tears. One man had since birth never had any distinct growth of hair anywhere on his body, and additionally was without a tooth in his head, with no sense of smell and almost no sense of taste. He had no apparent perspiration, and when working actively he was obliged to wet his clothes in order to moderate the heat of his body. He could sleep in wet clothes in a damp cellar without catching cold. There was some hair in the armpits and on the pubes, but only the slightest down on the scalp, and even that was absent from his skin. His maternal grandmother and uncle were similarly affected. He himself was the youngest of twenty-one children. One comfort to him was that he had never been ill, not even with stomach-ache or indigestion; though he was not able to chew food in the normal manner, he had never suffered dyspepsia in any form. He was married and had eight children. Two of his daughters were lacking in a number of the teeth they should have had, but they had the ordinary amount of hair. Congenital alopecia in women has meant that not only is the head completely bald, but there are no eyebrows or eyelashes. As with men, the condition can involve toothlessness and an inability to perspire. Partial alopecia in women has been known on occasion to be restricted to the genital area. One medical researcher recorded the case of a prostitute whose body was completely and naturally devoid of hair in the pubic region. ¶ Growth of pubic hair, like that of the beard, is of course governed by the development of the sexual hormones and the state of sexual maturity of the subject. But the biological clock within the body may be set before the actual onset of puberty. Artificial eunuchs, that is, men born with the normal testicular equipment but later castrated, do lose their beard growth to a degree but are not naturally devoid of pubic hair. Women whose ovaries are removed tend to develop extra facial

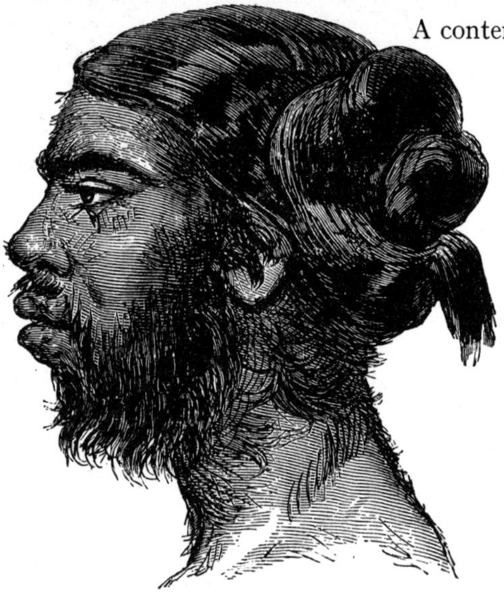

A contemporary engraving of Julia Patrana.

FACING

The 'Dog-Man' Lionel.

hair, and all women have this tendency after the menopause. ¶ Bearded women have never been an infrequent occurrence, and were medically recorded long before Victorian times. But it was in the nineteenth century, the peak period for the commercial exhibition of abnormality, that they became most widely known. Julia Pastrana, seen here in profile but in a less aggressive posture than in the previous portrait, has already been mentioned in connection with her pathetic love affair and the subsequent exploitation by her manager-widower. The presence of a beard on a woman does not necessarily imply any masculinization of her sentiments. In the *British Medical Journal* of 2 June 1894 Harris published a study of a number of bearded women, one of whom plaited her 8-inch beard (though her moustache did not grow to a length of more than an inch) and she 'exhibited a strong passion for the male sex', even at the age of sixty-four. The beard of one Kentucky lady was 15 inches long. ¶ One of the most famous exhibitors of the exaggerated development of facial and body hair was the 'Dog-Man' Lionel. Explorers among primitive people had long reported this condition, and their reasoning had been that it was more natural that primitive people, who are not provided with the artificial protection of copious clothing to shield them from the wind, should be supplied with an additional

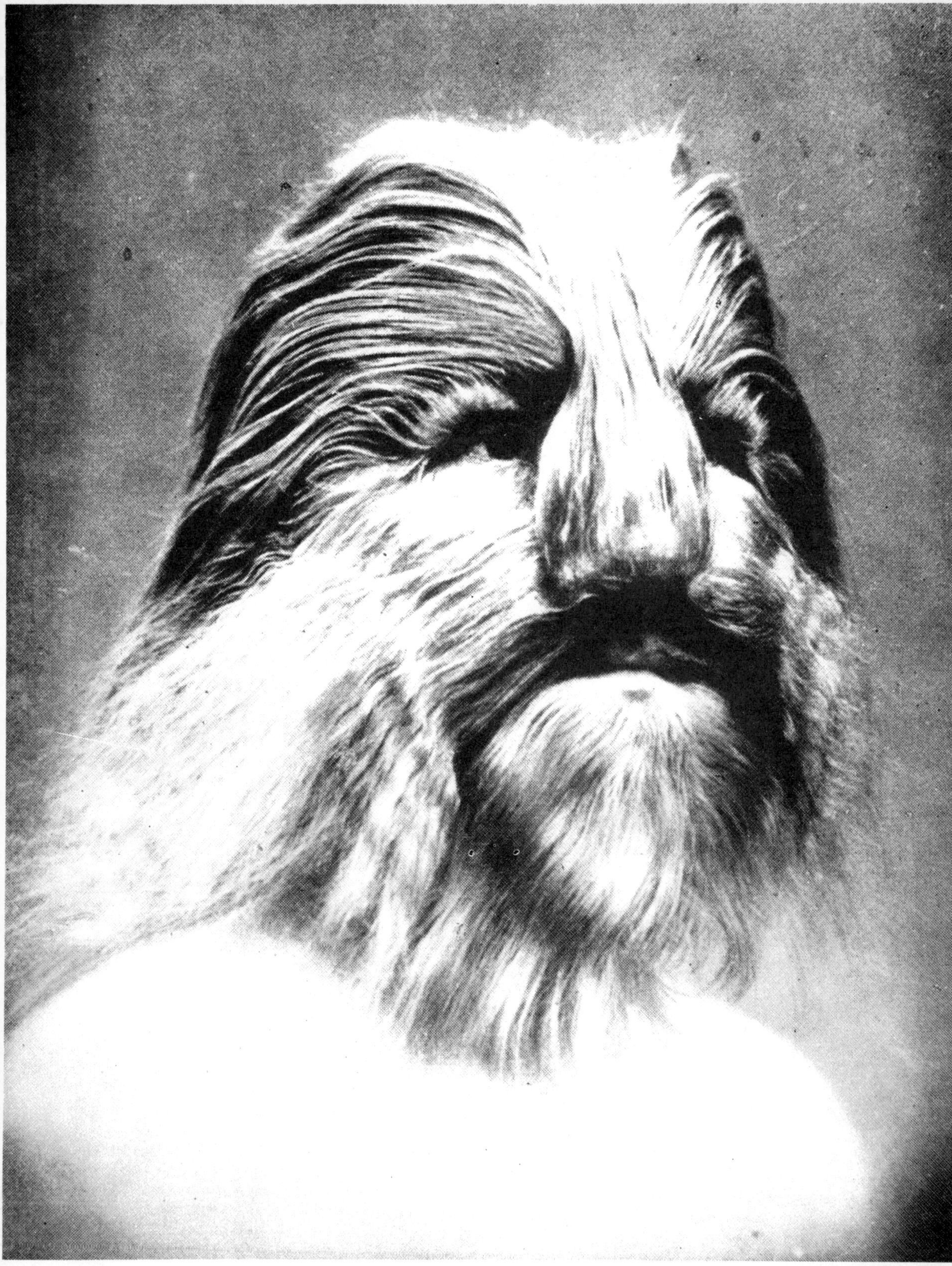

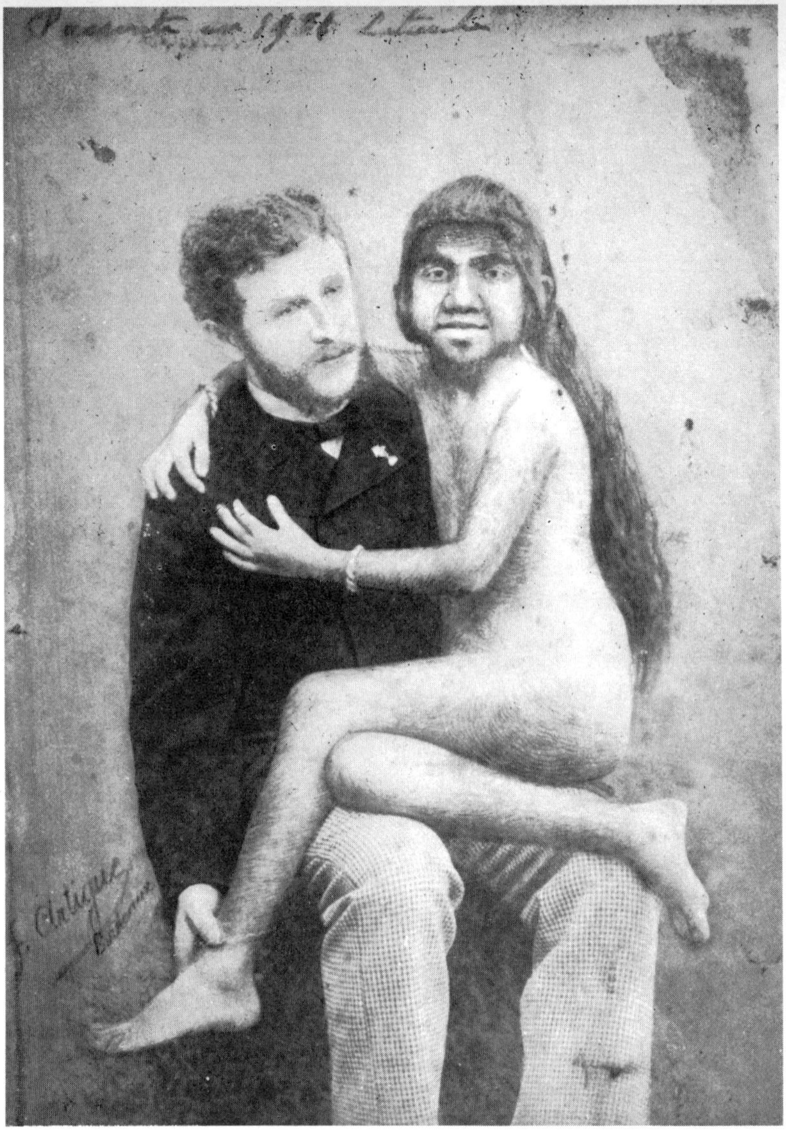

Dr George Shelley and the seven-year-old Krao.

hairy coat, like animals. In 1883 Dr George Shelly put on exhibition a seven-year-old girl called Krao who had been brought from Laos in Indo-China. According to the review *Nature* (12 May 1883), she was covered all over her body with stiff, straight black hair. Her jaws had a marked forward development. She had the faculty of projecting her lips to an extraordinary degree, like a chimpanzee, and when she did this she displayed a pout very characteristic of that animal. Her feet were extremely prehensile, and with them she could pick up the most delicate objects from the ground. Because of the abnormal powers of her prehensile lips and feet she was given the title of 'Darwin's missing link', but the anthropologist Keane carefully examined her and pronounced that in all respects she was a member of the genus *Homo sapiens*. Indeed, she had some skill with languages and could pronounce English reasonably well: a circumstance which, since Keane himself was an Englishman, in his opinion qualified her for full membership of the human race. Krao's family in Laos were also of a hairy nature, the explorer Bock having brought back photographs of them to demonstrate this. Keane maintained in *Nature* that the child was living proof of his theory that there existed in Laos a race of hairy people similar to the Hairy Ainus. ¶ The Ainus are a dying race, now found principally in the island of Hokkaido in Japan and in Sakhalin. They were probably among the aborigines of Japan, and the early history of the region tells of fierce conflicts with them. They are tall, strong, and very hairy. Their cheek-bones are high, their noses flat and broad, and their faces short. They are still primarily hunters and fishers. They have a peculiar religion, principally worshipping the bear, yet they pay no respect to the life of this animal. They kill and skin it without fear, and set up its head for veneration in their villages. They combine this worship, however, with belief in a Supreme Creating God and in the immortality of the soul. The Ainus differ in physique, language, and customs from all other Asiatic races, and they are generally considered to have originated from the Caucasus. They are no longer a pure civilization, having become almost intermingled with the Japanese. Basically, however, their facial characteristics are remarkably different, along with their propensity to hair, which is the reverse of the physical condition of the Japanese. ¶ A remarkable confirmation of the theory that the Hairy Ainus originated from the Caucasus is offered by the Caucasian gentleman of more than hirsute appearance who was another exhibit of considerable drawing power in the Victorian scene, and whose portrait is given here. ¶ Extreme hairiness can have a hereditary aspect, as is illustrated by the Burmese family who made a successful exhibition tour towards the end of the Victorian age. From a nearby locality came Jo-Jo,

Extreme hirsuitness in a White Russian.

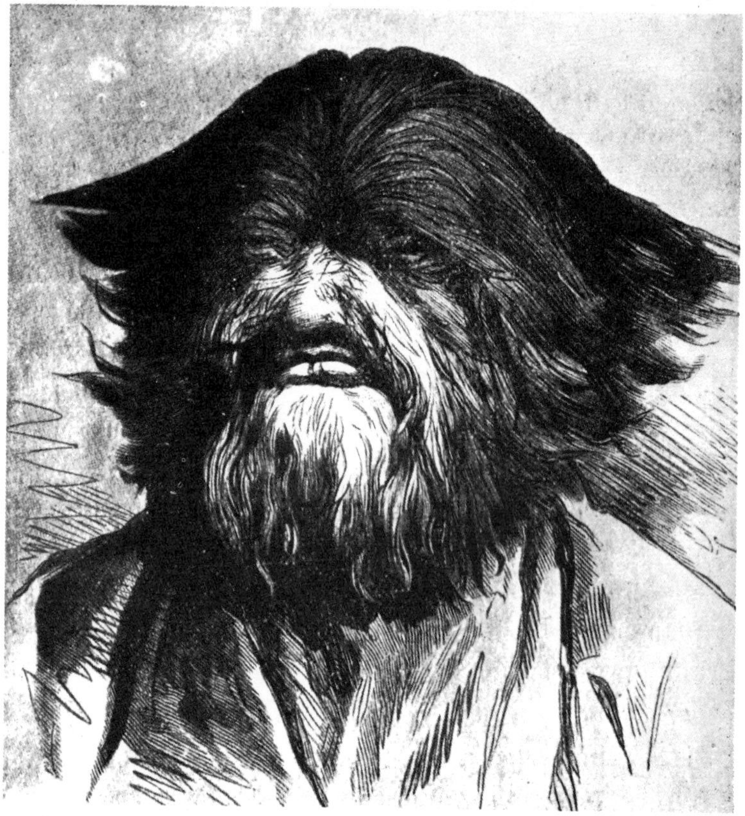

Two examples of extreme hirsuties in a Burmese family.

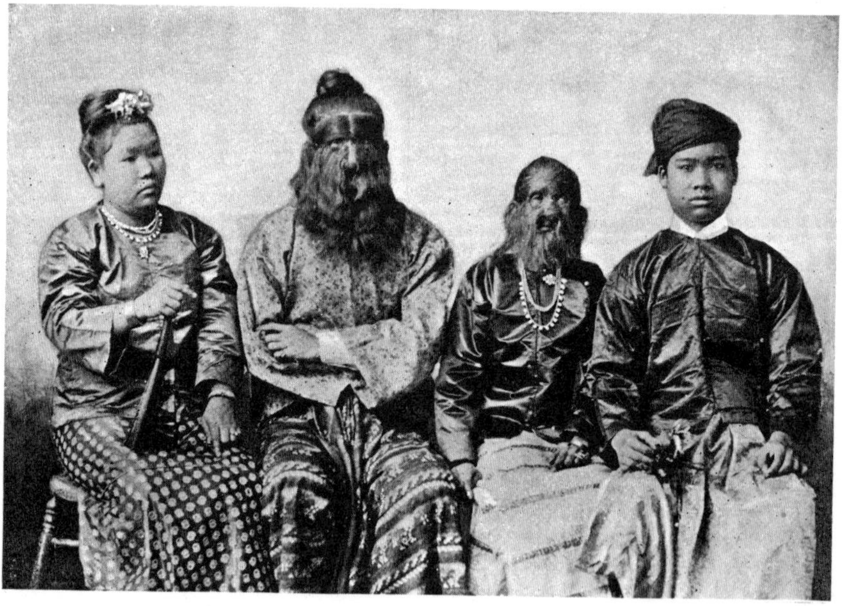

'the Dog-Faced Boy', whose face was confidently said to be 'truly that of a Skye-terrier'. ¶ Many cases of abnormal growth of hair are classified as naevus pilosus, or an exaggerated instance of the hairy mole which affects many people. Sometimes a complete limb can be covered with hair originating from such a mole. The condition can cover a large part of the body, sometimes up to a quarter of the skin area. In other cases it occurs quite locally, and it has been only the bizarre positioning of this appendage that has prompted the exhibition of the subject. If the hair occurs in the place that might be taken by a tail it affords more general amusement than elsewhere. Dufour mentioned in the Paris *Archives générales de médicine* a young man of twenty whose sacral region (above the cleft in the buttocks) contained a tuft of hair as long and black, thick, and pliant as the hair of the head. Particularly remarkable in this case was the fact that the skin from which the hair grew was as fine and white as on the rest of the body, with no visible darkening as in the hairy mole more commonly met. Another exhibit well known to Victorians was 'the Woman with the Mane', a lady who had growing from the centre of her back between the shoulders a convincing 'mane' of long dark hair which medical observers concluded came from a naevus pilosus. ¶ Normally situated hair growing to an exaggerated length becomes an object of curiosity in the case of a man with a long beard, and an object of sheer envy in that of a woman with luxuriant hair. Dr Erasmus Wilson of London recorded the case of a thirty-eight-year-old woman whom he had seen whose hair was 5 feet 5 inches long. Leonard of Philadelphia gave the relevant vital statistic of a man whose beard trailed on the ground when he stood upright, and measured 7 feet 4 inches. The greatest commercial exploitation of long hair occurred in the case of the Seven Sutherland Sisters, very famous in Victoria's day, all of whom had hair which touched the ground. They were immediately cornered by the proprietors of a hair tonic and their communal photographs were constantly displayed in newspaper advertisements declaring that this luxuriant growth was entirely due to the application of Thatcho, the great specific for thinning

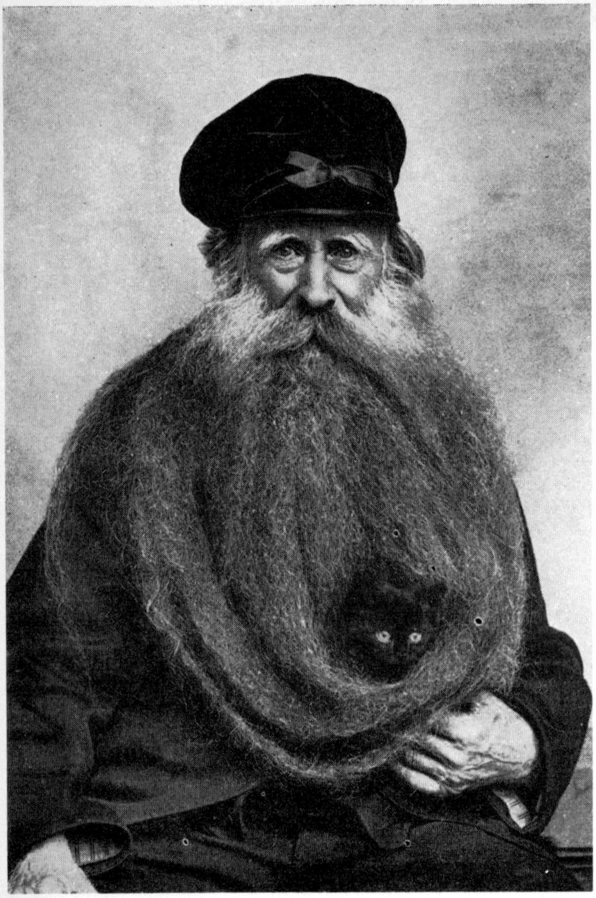

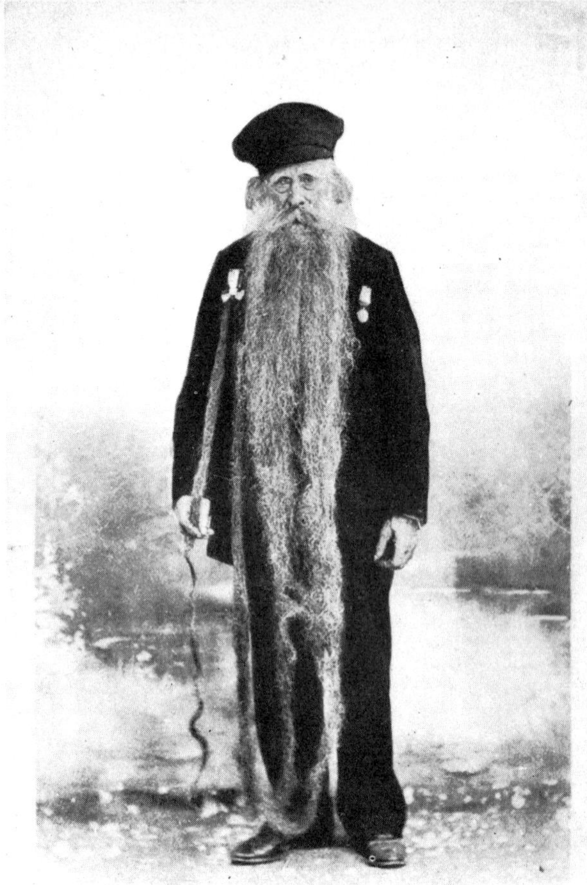

Louis Coulon whose beard was 11 feet long.

hair. ¶ Certainly no candidate for Thatcho was Louis Coulon, portrayed with the medals he doubtless earned, who sported a beard no less than 11 feet long – which, naturally, he had to drape up and down around his lapels when he walked, always careful not to obscure those medals. In his domestic moments he used to curl his beard up and put the cat to sleep in the nest. But even Louis was floored by the venerable Jules Dumont, a property-owner of northern France. And what a property he owned. At the age of fifty-five his beard measured 12 feet in length, and, as will be obvious from his portrait, he could only display it to best advantage by walking backwards, like a Victorian debutante managing her train when leaving the presence of her beloved Queen. ¶ Individually, the Sutherland Sisters were bested by a rival named Miss Owens, whose hair was longer even than her skirts (even in those days) and measured at full stretch 8 feet

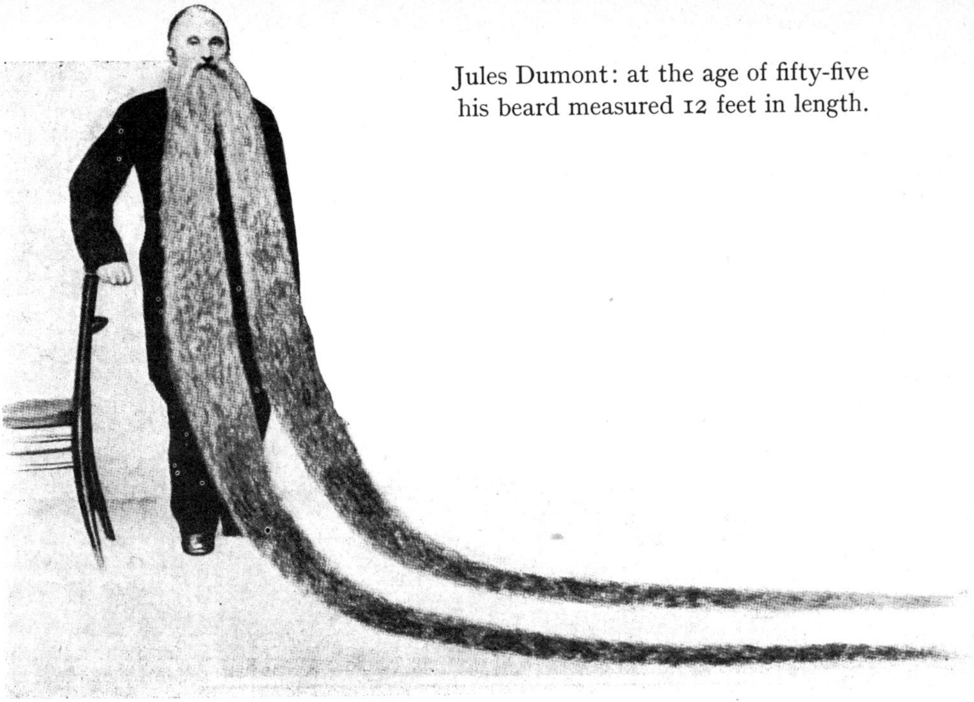

Jules Dumont: at the age of fifty-five his beard measured 12 feet in length.

3 inches. As can be seen, there was a natural curl in the hair which took up some of the surplus. To complete the record with an earlier winner, it may be recounted that the chronicles hold the details of a woman whose pubic hair hung down to her knees, a condition which provoked the composition of a merry song much performed in football changing-rooms. And in the animal world the record growth of horse-hair is held by a Percheron written up in *Nature* (9 January 1892) whose mane measured 13 feet and whose tail was almost 10 feet long. ¶ Tufts of different-coloured hair, always fashionable with women as some prevaricating concession to going grey, have occurred even in new-born infants, which have sometimes been delivered with tufts (not down) on their heads which are perfectly white in colour. Premature blanching of the hair was put down in Victorian times to a variety of causes which included 'over-indulgence in the sexual appetite' and 'mercurial courses too frequently repeated' (the then common treatment for venereal diseases) as well as paroxysms of rage, the receipt of unexpected unwelcome news, and the sudden impact of anxiety which is still

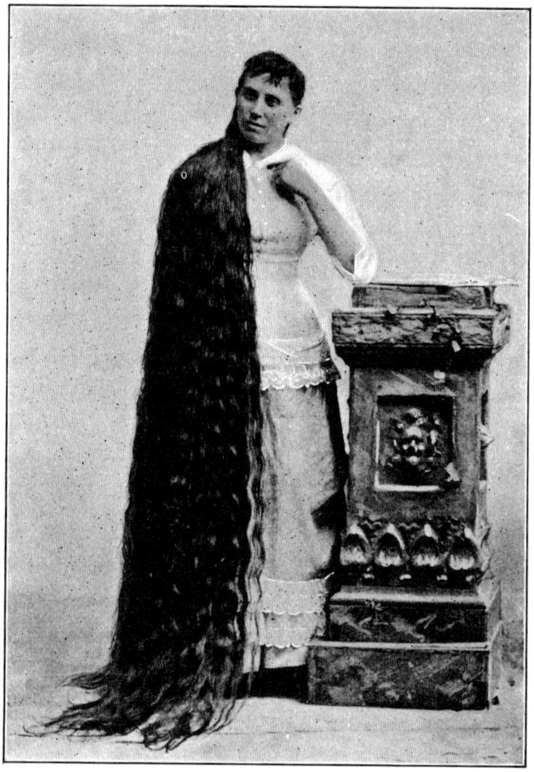

Example of excessive growth of hair.

popularly considered as a cause. ¶ It has long been accepted that worry or fear, or some other violent emotion, can cause the hair to change colour suddenly. Sometimes medical observation recorded a peculiar physical mutation accompanying and possibly causing the condition. Landois in Paris had a patient admitted to hospital with delirium tremens who for four days, until his condition improved, was tormented by terrifying pictures of the imagination. On the third night the patient's head and beard, formerly blond, became grey. Landois made a careful examination and showed that the pigment contents of the hair were unchanged, which led him to believe that the white colour was solely due to the excessive development of air bubbles in the shafts of the hair. There are many historical records of hair 'turning white in a night'. The best authenticated as to colour, but not as to the speed of the change, was the alteration in the colouring of Marie Antoinette, the queen of Louis XVI, who went white to the guillotine at the age of thirty-eight in 1793 during the excesses of the French Revolution. It was said to be grief rather than fear which had caused the change, although she had long been imprisoned. The grief was for her husband, who had been guillotined nine months earlier. ¶ The theory that air bubbles in the hair and scalp are a contributory cause of suddenly changed colour was repeated in a symposium on this subject printed in *Science* (3 October 1890). A man who had gone suddenly white through business worries was examined, and the microscope showed a great many air-vesicles, both in the medullary substance ('marrow') and between this and the outer surface of the hair shafts. A case of a man who had been 'scared white' in an instant was examined, and the possible additional cause of sickness was considered. The patient was a man of thirty who while working in a mining camp had become ill and had been left alone in the camp sleeping. He woke up and found a grizzly bear standing over him. The consequence, from whatever cause, was that his hair went completely white. Another case mentioned was that of a man aged twenty-three who was gambling in California. He staked his entire savings of eleven hundred dollars on the turn of a card and was under tremendous nervous excitement while the cards were being dealt. 'The next day his hair was perfectly white.' This account peevishly omits the climax of the story. Did the gambler win or lose? It would have been interesting to have a record of a man who was not 'scared white' but shocked white through joy. The condition of previous nervous excitement would hold, of course, for either eventuality. ¶ Cases have been recorded where, for instance, a healthy brunette girl of eighteen found her eyelashes turned white in a week. It has been known for the eyelashes to become white after smallpox, and for eyebrows and eyelashes to lose colour as a result of neuralgia of the trigeminal nerves – those nerves of the cranium which affect the skin and flesh of the face, and the tongue and teeth. ¶ Often a sudden whitening of the hair as a result of sickness will reverse itself when health is regained. It is thought that particular diseases or conditions can affect the pigment-forming function of the melanin supply. One woman went completely white during the course of a malignant fever, but seven days later the colour of the hair was completely restored. Some people even change their hair to white in winter and dark in summer, like the stoat, which is reddish-brown in summer and changes to become the white ermine in winter. Other people have been known to lose their hair during a sickness and on recovery to grow new hair of a completely different colour – most often bright red. Fair hair has lost its colour during sickness and changed to tawny red, but the effect has been reversible with the regainment of health. Crocker of Edinburgh recorded the case of an epileptic girl of a manic-depressive type whose hair was blonde when she was in a state of stupor but changed to bright red at times of manic excitement. The change of colour took place in the course of two or three days, and the colour stayed for about a week in the case of the red tint. The pale hairs had more air-spaces than the darker ones. ¶ Hair can change colour because of chemicals in the environment, particularly in industry. Blue hair was seen among workers in the Victorian cobalt mines and indigo works, green hair among copper smelters, and deep red-brown hair among the handlers of crude aniline, the dye which was over-exploited at that time. Chemical lotions which are now no longer used also carried their dangers. People who had been prescribed chrysarobin applications for the scalp found their hair going purple if they washed it, owing to the alkaline action of the soap on the lotion. ¶ The principal anomalies of the nails are their entire absence, their exaggerated growth, or their displacement. Some persons are born with finger-nails and toe-nails either very rudimentary or completely absent. Others sport nails of great length or thickness. In the nineteenth century the Chinese nobility – much more familiar to the empire-building Victorians than the mandarin-commissars are to Westerners today – allowed their finger-nails to grow to great length and spent much time in the care of them. The horror stories of sinister Chinese villains which graduated into the Edwardian sagas of Dr Fu Manchu were not entirely fanciful. Some savage tribes were discovered possessing long and thick nails resembling the claws of a beast, and they were observed to use them in the same way as the lower animals. A collection of monstrous nails was preserved in the Académie des Sciences of Paris. The largest was a left great toe-nail which from its extremity to its root measured $4\frac{3}{4}$ inches. The layers of which it was made up were placed one over the other at a remove, like the tiles on a roof but reversed. This nail and several of the others were of unequal thickness and were variously curved, probably on account of the pressure of the boot or of the neighbouring digits. An earlier record mentions the nails of a girl of twenty, which grew to such a size that the finger-nails were 5 inches long. They were composed of several layers. These nails fell off at the end of four months, and were succeeded by others. There were also horny layers on the knees, shoulders, and elbows which bore a resemblance to talons rather than nails. They were sensitive only at the point of insertion into the skin. Various other parts of the body, particularly the backs of the hands, presented these horny productions. One of them was 4 inches long. The whole condition of this horny growth seems to have occurred after the patient had been stricken with smallpox. ¶ Teeth have their peculiarities of incidence also. Many instances have been recorded of children born with several teeth already erupted. King Richard III was one of the historical figures reputed to have been born with this condition. It did not necessarily mean that the subject was exhibiting remarkable strength, since several of the children born with this condition died very early. The maximum number of teeth recorded at birth seems to be nine, reported in the *American Journal of Obstetrics.* ¶ A number of instances of triple dentition, the development of a third set of teeth, were recorded. There is an account of a country labourer who had lost all his teeth by the time he was sixty, but six months later was cheered by the sprouting of a new set. One old woman was declared to have developed twelve fresh molars at the age of ninety-eight. There is one unique record of the appearance of a fourth set of teeth. They were presented to a woman who had a third set when she was forty-seven; but after

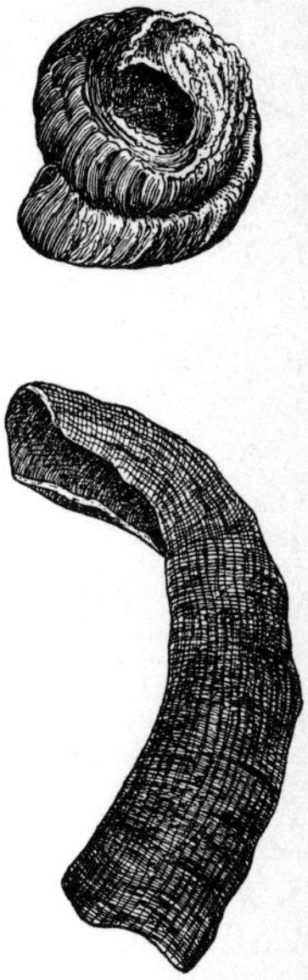

Deformed toe-nails.

energetic use these finally fell out. The fourth set came when she was sixty-seven, and these were apparently of a more reliable nature, for she was still making do with the survivors when she was ninety. ¶ Permanent toothlessness has already been noted as one of the accompaniments of hairlessness. Many cases where this occurs are also connected with a lack of the senses of smell and taste. Excessive dentition is far more common. Most often this is noticed by the arrival of individual supernumerary teeth, but occasionally they arrive in a series such as the development of four canines above the usual equipment. Many persons have the supernumerary teeth parallel with their neighbours, forming the beginnings of a double row. In 1895 Costa reported in the *Gazeta medica da Bahia* a case in which there were five canine teeth in the upper jaw, two placed laterally on either side, and one on the right side behind the other two. The patient was twenty-six years old, well developed and in good health. ¶ In some cases there is fusion of teeth. In the Musée de l'École Dentaire de Paris there are several milk teeth, of both the upper and lower jaw, which are fused together. One case is cited of two complete rows of teeth fused in the upper jaw, and there is even a report of three rows of teeth similarly merged. ¶ Perhaps the most curious anomaly of teeth is that in which they are found in abnormal positions – in the nose or the palate, or under the tongue. Dr Dave, a Norwegian doctor, reporting to the Medical Society in Christiana (now Oslo) in 1895, showed a tooth removed from the nose of a woman of fifty-three. She had consulted him for ear trouble, and the tooth was found accidentally during the routine examination. It was easily removed, since it was situated in a small depression in the nasal cavity. This patient had all her teeth, placed somewhat far from each other. The tooth resembled a milk canine and its root was imperfect. Dr Dave suggested that before birth part of the mucous membrane of the mouth with its tooth-germ had become impacted between the upper jaw and the premaxillary bone and thus had become cut off from the cavity of the mouth. In the subsequent discussion another doctor rejected this theory and suggested that the abnormality was due to an inversion, by development in the wrong direction, which had caused the tooth to grow upwards into the nose. ¶ Dr Gould made the suggestion – following an observation that it was not rare to see teeth, generally canine, make their eruption from the vault of the palate – that these teeth are not generally supernumerary, but are examples of deviation from the normal position. An undoubted deviation was described in 1887 by Dr Carver, who reported the case of a child who had a tooth growing from the lower right eyelid. ¶ The most serious anomalies of the head are found in those monsters born without a brain. They do not survive for subsequent examination and discussion; the longest known period for which they have been kept alive is eight days. Almost as doomed are those creatures born without a cerebellum, the outgrowth from the back of the brain which controls movement. This condition, particularly when it is a case of partial lack of function rather than the entire loss, is not necessarily fatal but is none the less miserable. Patients can live for many years. In 1880 Fraser reported a brother and sister, then aged twenty and thirty, who had from birth exhibited defective development of the cerebellum. They lacked the power of co-ordination and walked with a drunken, staggering gait. They could not touch the nose with the finger when their eyes were shut – an interesting exercise which is still used as an unofficial test of drunkenness, and which formerly was part of the police surgeon's book before the introduction of the breathalyser. Though the defect seemed to have been due to some hereditary cause, the parents of these two were perfectly healthy, as were the rest of their children. The longest case of survival of a human born with no cerebellum recorded in the Victorian age is eleven years. This was a French girl, who previously had exhibited all the signs of non-co-ordination mentioned above. ¶ Victorian scientists were intrigued by an experiment from Ann Arbor, Michigan, reported in 1880 in *Physician and Surgeon*, which, they thought, reinforced the argument that the brain is not the sole organ of the mind, but there is some other location of the will and the senses, even in lower animals. A rooster cock had been well-nigh decapitated by the stroke of a knife. 'The knife had severed the larynx and removed the whole mass of the cerebrum [the larger part of the brain], leaving the inner aspect and base of the skull exposed. The cerebrum was partly removed; the external auditory meatus [ear cavity] was preserved. Immediately after the decapitation the rooster was left to its supposed death struggles, but it ran headless to the barn, where it was secured and subsequently fed by pushing corn down its esophagus [gullet], and allowing water to trickle into this tube from the spout of an oil-can. The phenomena exhibited by the rooster were quite interesting. It made all the motions of pecking, strutted about, flapped its wings, attempted to crow, but, of course, without making any sound. It exhibited no signs of incoordination, but did not seem to hear. A ludicrous exhibition was the absurd, sidelong *pas seul* made toward the hens.' ¶ Diminution in the volume of the head is called microcephaly. A small head generally entails a small brain, but, though it seems logical, it is not necessarily correct to deduce from this fact that the subject has small intelligence. The superior intelligence of some dwarfs (though dwarfs do not generally have abnormally small heads) will be discussed in a later chapter. The record case of microcephaly was an individual exhibited as 'the Bird-Man' who was examined by Lombroso. Cesare Lombroso was one of the great intellectual heroes of the Victorians. In 1862 at the age of only twenty-six he was professor of psychiatry at Pavia University and he then became director of the Pesaro lunatic asylum. He gradually followed his bent to become a criminologist, and was appointed professor of forensic medicine, and later professor of criminal anthropology, at Turin. He specialized in theories of the responsibility or irresponsibility of criminals, which he based on their physical and and psychical characteristics. In particular he attempted to establish the existence of criminal types who could be judged by the shape of the head (hence his interest in microcephaly). He maintained that criminality was an inborn characteristic which was associated with certain physical signs of degeneracy – and these could be recognized. The characteristics he nominated included a receding forehead, a small cranium, and projecting ears. Later in his life – and Lombroso outlived Victoria – there were many critics of his work. One of the principals in the opposite camp was the English Dr Goring, an officer in the prison service, who showed that Lombroso's so-called stigmata of degeneracy were found with equal frequency amongst non-criminal persons. This came as a great relief to all those with ears sticking out who had previously found themselves suspect whenever they wandered into a bank. Lombroso's obvious failing, as a scientific researcher in a difficult new field, was that he did not maintain a control group – that is, a group of persons, preferably chosen at random, some of whom would be normal and some of whom, on statistical probabilities, ought to be abnormal – with whom he could contrast his research findings. But the Victorians were deeply impressed by Lombroso, and although his views are no longer fervently accepted he is recognized as the first criminologist to break away from a purely moral attitude to crime and to try to discover its causes by scientific investigation. ¶ Lombroso's 'Bird-Man' had a cranial capacity of only 390 cubic centimetres, or about two-thirds of a pint. A runner-up who also came to Lombroso's attention as 'the Rabbit-Man' was only slightly larger in the skull. Microcephaly was found geographically among some of the Asian peoples and among the population of the Caribbean. It was also noted among the ancient Aztecs, not only from the ancient portraits, but in the skulls dug up. For this reason, when two people with extremely receding foreheads were discovered by show business and put on exhibition, they were billed as 'the Aztec Children'. They were actually a man and a woman, Maximo and Bartola, and they made a living out of their criminal appearance for twenty-five years. As will be seen from the portrait of the 'Aztec' man, the receding forehead in their profile gave them a marked resemblance to the heads on the bas-reliefs found in ancient Aztec temples in Mexico. Their facial angle was about 45° and they had jutting lips and little or no chin. They wore their hair in an enormous bunch to magnify their deformity. In addition, the 'Aztecs' were of very short stature. They were not, of course, real Aztecs, although

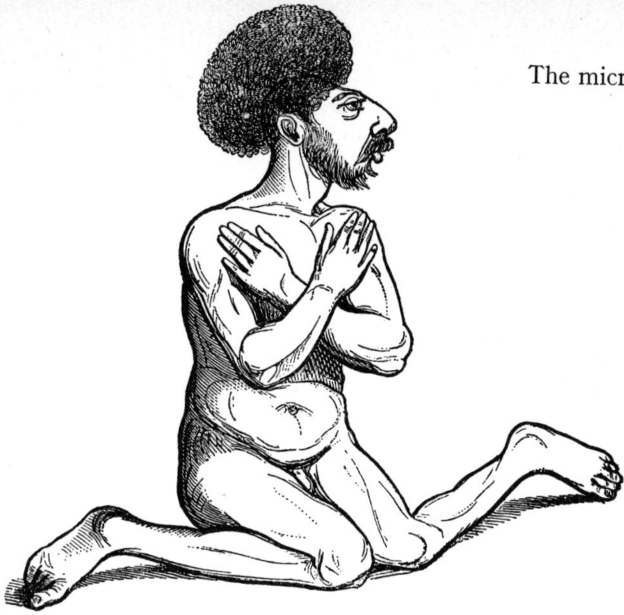

The microcephalic 'Aztec man'.

there could possibly have been some sort of throwback through heredity. They were born in Central America, and were thought to be possibly half-Indian and half-Negro. Their intelligence rating would have gratified Lombroso, for they were said to be little better than idiots. What they thought, after being hauled out of their birthplace and toted around a country they did not understand to demonstrate an ancient likeness they did not appreciate, would have been worth a scientific record, whether from a criminologist or any other anthropologist. The only certainty is that, since they did not know what was going on, they did not count, nor equitably share, the gate-money that was taken for the privilege of gaping at them. ¶ Another microcephalic young man was on the American circuit and known as 'the Mexican Wild Boy'. Unlike the 'Aztecs' he was of normal stature, and it is clear that when he was not seen in profile the smallness of his skull was far less noticeable. The receding forehead of this type must make for a certain diminution in the maturing development of the original brain. Microcephaly has been observed to be associated with mental retardation and the arrested development of the rest of the body. The scientific explanation then given was that ossification of the fontanelles

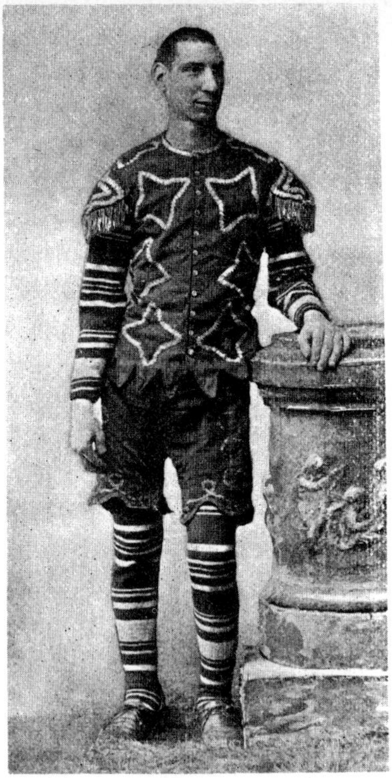

A microcephalic boy.

(premature bony hardening of the soft spaces partitioning the skull of an infant) would necessarily prevent full development of the brain. In Victorian days some tribes of American Indians still voluntarily sought a kind of artificial microcephaly by the practice of head-binding, analogous to the contemporary Chinese custom of binding the feet of women, which produced its own style of hideous deformity. ¶ When the head is abnormally large, but roughly in fair proportion compared with a normal head, the condition is called macrocephaly. One of the most striking examples recorded was of a male whose head began to enlarge at the age of seven. Twenty years later it measured over 37 inches in circumference, and was 15 inches high. No other part of the man's body was affected or increased abnormally. His voice was of a normal timbre and he was a very intelligent person. The subject died of apoplexy at the age of thirty. ¶ A locked cabinet in the Natural History Museum of Marseilles used to contain the skull of a man named Borghini, whose head measured 3 feet in circumference and was a foot in height. In later years – he died when he was past fifty – he could not maintain the weight of his head, and he carried a cushion on each shoulder to prop it up. Another Marseillais with the same condition never lay on a bed for thirty years, since his head projected downwards beyond his body in that position, and he passed his nights in a chair, not often sleeping but reading or writing. He ate only once in twenty-four or thirty hours, never warmed himself, and never used warm water. He was reputed to have been a man of great intelligence and of an encyclopaedic knowledge commensurate with all those nights spent reading. Victorians celebrated one Englishman, James Cardinal, whose head was a mere $32\frac{1}{2}$ inches round. The largest healthy brains on record are roughly 25 per cent larger than the average. This is a peculiarly restricted league in which to notch any record, since 'the best people' (which may include the most intelligent) do not normally assign their brains for weighing after death. In England it was only the criminals hanged at Tyburn and Newgate who underwent the indignity of compulsory dissection – and certainly none of them qualified for the largest brain. ¶ Those who did enter the record-book were all contemporary Victorians, though one was French, one English, and one American. The winner was the Frenchman Baron Cuvier, with $64\frac{1}{3}$ oz. (The average male brain weighs 50 oz., the average female brain 45 oz.) Cuvier was an enthusiast who highly approved of his own dissection, though he gave no previous hint that he had a marginal hope of scooping the prize. He was certainly a fine-looking man with a remarkable head. He began as an anatomist who re-classified the invertebrate animals, published unparalleled research on the fossils of quadrupeds, re-organized education throughout the whole of the Napoleonic empire, and finally wrote the standard work on zoology. He was in some ways a reactionary, and became a bitter opponent of the dawning theory of evolution; but at least he was forward-looking enough to permit the dissection of his skull. The runner-up in the weighty brain contest was Daniel Webster, who ran for the presidency of the United States (had he been successful, his inaugural year would have coincided with the accession of Queen Victoria). His brain weighed $63\frac{3}{4}$ oz., which was then considered

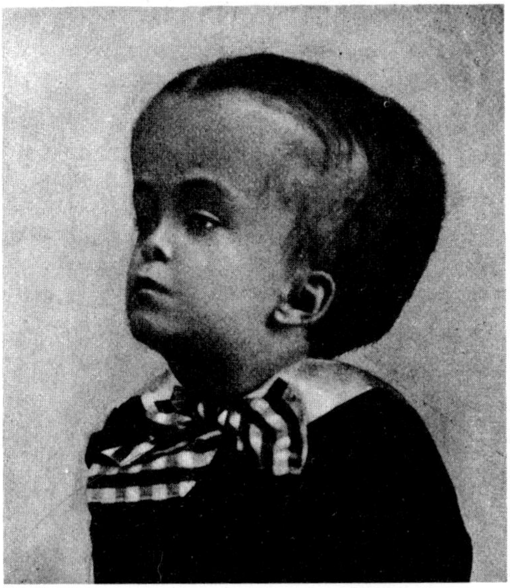

A hydrocephalic child.

only as remarkable as it ought to be, since his head was 23¾ inches in circumference. The third in line was John Abercrombie, an Aberdeen surgeon who became an inspiring teacher of pathological anatomy, and had the courage of his convictions when the time came for his own pathological anatomizing. His brain weighed 63 oz. Two historical figures who had abnormally heavy brains were Byron and Cromwell, but both organs showed marked evidence of disease. ¶ When the increase in the natural volume of the skull is caused by an excess of serous fluid, the anomaly is known as hydrocephaly, which has always been known popularly as 'water on the brain'. In this condition there is usually no change in the size of the brain structure itself, but often the cranial bones are rent asunder. The heads of infants even have been measured at up to 43 inches in circumference. The child illustrated had a head circumference of 36 inches at the age of six. Hydrocephalics do live, and the Victorians would pay to see them on exhibition. ¶ Other abnormalities of the head have included complete absence of the lower jaw-bone, exaggerated prominence of both jaw-bones (known as prognathism), and congenital absence of the nose: a rare phenomenon. Exaggeration in the volume of the nose is more frequent, and has been a source

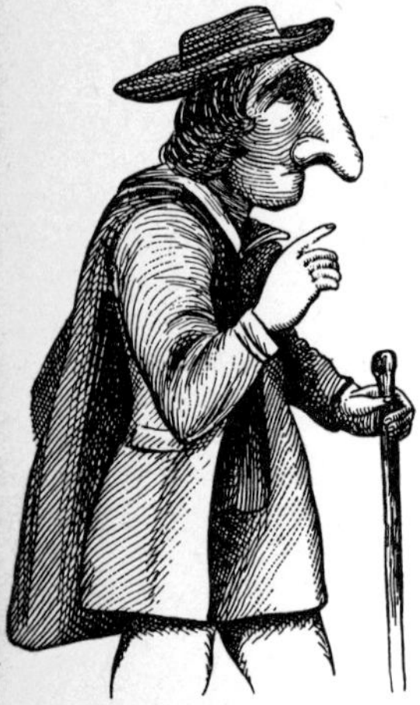

Thomas Wedders.

of amusement to all but the unfortunate subject since long before Cyrano de Bergerac. One of the most gigantic noses recorded belonged to the Yorkshireman Thomas Wadhouse (usually pronounced and spelt Wedders), whose nose was 7½ inches long and, though drawn by an artist before the age of photography, is considered to be reasonably accurately reproduced in the accompanying illustration. ¶ A number of historical celebrities, including William of Orange, have had extremely short noses, and in Victorian days 'button noses' were considered no more a sign of beauty than great eagle's conks. There have been cases of people with two noses, most often due to a congenital division of the nose, but occasionally displaying a supernumerary nose, sometimes near the eye, through which air passes. Anomalies of the mouth known to the nineteenth century were concerned with its being either too big or too small. There was a record from Göttingen in the *Bibliothek für die Chirurgie* of a boy aged seventeen with a mouth 6½ inches across. His mother claimed that the boy was born with his foot in his mouth, and in fact attributed the size of the mouth to this occurrence. The Negro races were considered to be noted for their large mouths, and a Negro called Black Diamond who went on show in Philadelphia could put both his fists into his mouth together. Congenital macrostoma, that is, the affliction of being born with an abnormally large mouth, may be produced by lateral fissures extending on both sides, or can be restricted to one side, where a lateral fissure may be accompanied by a fistula of Stensen's duct, that is, an opening up of the normally covered cavity leading from the mouth to the salivary gland which opens opposite the first top molar tooth. ¶ The Victorians knew of a few cases in which the mouth was so small or ill-defined as not to admit any supply of food. The most striking anomalies of the lips – apart from harelip, which doctors were then not generally equipped to deal with – occurred from such unfortunate conditions as elephantiasis of the face leading to exaggerated growth of the upper lip. Elephantiasis is a parasitic disease of the lymphatic vessels, those cavities secreting lymph, which is a part of blood plasma. The disease

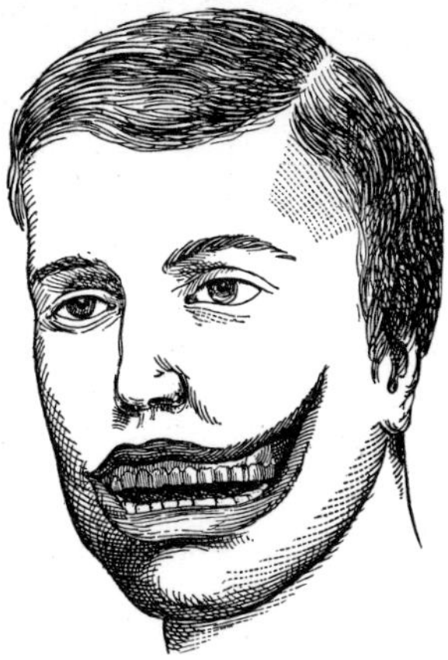

Deformitites in
the size of the mouth.

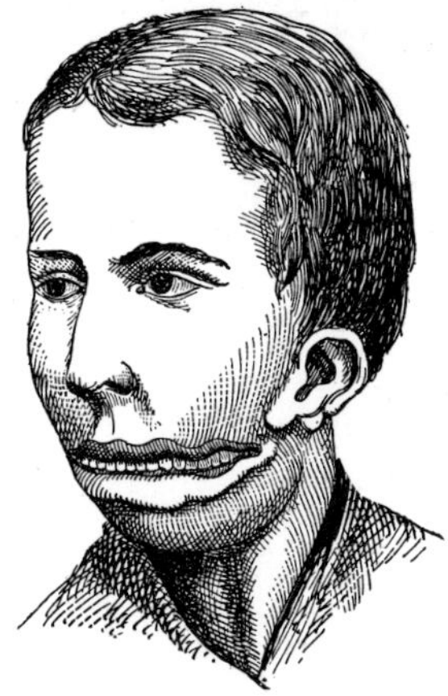

causes great enlargement of the part affected, the skin of which thickens until it resembles an elephant's hide. Cases sometimes occurred where the tongue was completely absent from birth, and at least one case was reported where the tongue was lost after an attack of smallpox. Absence of the tongue did not necessarily make speaking, tasting, or swallowing impossible. Tricks done with the tongue had to be of some complexity before they became classified as 'abnormal mobility of the tongue', but three doctors chronicled the ability of a patient to project the tongue into the nasopharynx, the space between the rear nostrils, the base of the skull, the soft palate, and the top of the oesophagus. Occasional cases of persons with forked tongues were noticed. Some people had an abnormal growth of tongue. Fournier, in a study of the tongue, mentioned a juggler with a tongue so long that he could extrude it 6 inches from his mouth. He spoke also of a woman in Berlin with an extremely long tongue which was 'thinner than that of a cat. When she laughed it hung over her teeth like a curtain, and was always extremely cold to the touch.' Fournier also described a man with a very long neck who could touch his tongue to his chest without bending his head. ¶ Examples have been known of people with either no uvula or a double uvula. More interest was taken in cases of a double epiglottis, the flap of cartilage and mucous membrane which is closed while swallowing by having the glottis (or top of the windpipe) pushed against it. The glottis is also the division between the vocal chords, and duplication of the epiglottis can lead to some very special vocal effects. In the *British Medical Journal* of 1880 French described a professional singer and contortionist aged thirty who had become the possessor of an extra voice when he was sixteen. In high and falsetto tones he could run the scale from A to F in an upper and lower range. The compass of his low voice was so small that he could not reach the high notes of any song with it, and in singing he only used it to break in on the falsetto and produce a sensation. He was able to produce these notes because he had a double epiglottis. In the *Archives of Laryngology* (1 January 1882) Roe described a young lady who could whistle at will with the lower part of her throat without the aid of her lips. Examination of her larynx showed that the fundamental tones were produced by vibrations of the edges of the vocal chords, and the modifications were effected by a minute adjustment of the bands regulating the opening of the larynx above the chord, pressing firmly down on the lower cavity to form a damper which prevented the vibration of the chords except in their middle third. Fascinated by the ability of a woman singer to produce the highest notes and to display an extraordinary compass of voice, a specialist made an examination which showed that she had an unusual development of the larynx which enabled her to throw into vibration, and at different speeds, either the entire length of the vocal chords or only a part of the length. She had remarkable control of the muscles regulating the division and modification of the resonant cavities (resonance is produced by the varied use of the cavities of the larynx, the pharynx, the mouth, and the nostrils). This singer had a forked uvula and the two divisions sometimes operated independently. She also used the epiglottis to separate the cavities of the pharynx (the muscularly controlled sac at the back of the mouth) which gave an unusual resonance to her highest notes. ¶ Complete absence of the eyes is rare. Occasionally a cyclops is born – an infant with one single central eye – but one has never been known to survive. Four-eyed humans have been mentioned from time to time in the records, and in 1895 there was a report from Paris of a child born with eyes in the top of its head. Differences in the colour of the two eyes are so frequent that they have not been considered worth special chronicling. ¶ Complete absence of both external ears is also considered rare. Extra ears very near the normal auricle are on the contrary comparatively common and even in the nineteenth century presented no problem in early amputation. In one nineteenth-century survey of 50,000 children 33 were mentioned as having supernumerary auricles (external ear formations) generally placed near the tragus, the little eminence just inside the normal external ear. They were removed with no unpleasant after-effects. Supernumerary ears are sometimes hereditarily linked with other supernumerary members. There was one report of a man who had an extra nipple on his chest, and three of his five children were born with supernumerary ears. Occasionally, however, an extra ear was found far from the normal site, often on the neck. An 1870 report in the *British Medical Journal* gave a history which would not be accepted without great reservations nowadays. It mentioned the birth of a child with two perfect ears, but three extra ones on the right of the face and two extra on the left, and attributed the abnormality to the fact that before birth the mother had been frightened by the sight of a boy with hideous contractions in the neck. ¶ In some people who amused the Victorians there was an excessive development of the muscles of the ear, which enabled them to move their ears about in a manner similar to animals. Others had a natural perforation in the ear drum, so that they could blow tobacco smoke from the ear. One man was cited who could smoke a whole cigar without losing any smoke, since he made it leave by his mouth, nose, or ears. ¶ People born without limbs, as the result either of amputation within the womb or of embryonic malformation, were less well-known to the Victorians than, unhappily, they are today since the tragic thalidomide disaster. That they still have the possibility of physical grace is shown by the picture of Violetta, 'the Trunk-Woman'. More often there is a serious deficiency in the limbs. A celebrated French painter in Victorian times was Caesar Ducornet,

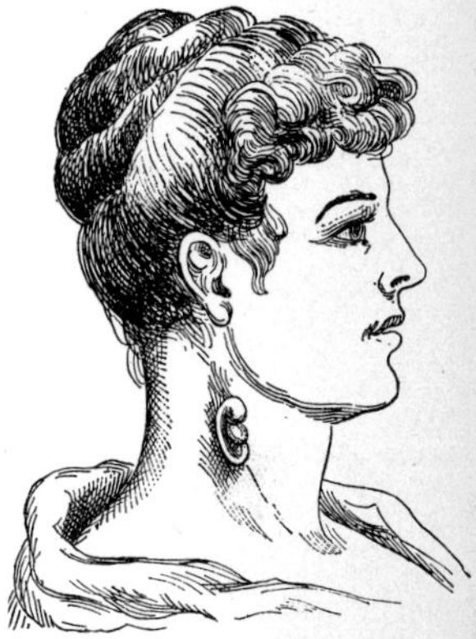

Supernumerary auricle in the neck.

Harvey Leach.

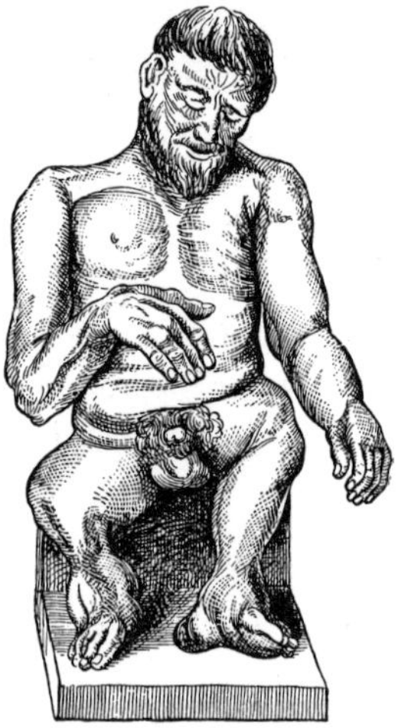

Violetta, the 'Trunk-Woman', had much physical grace.

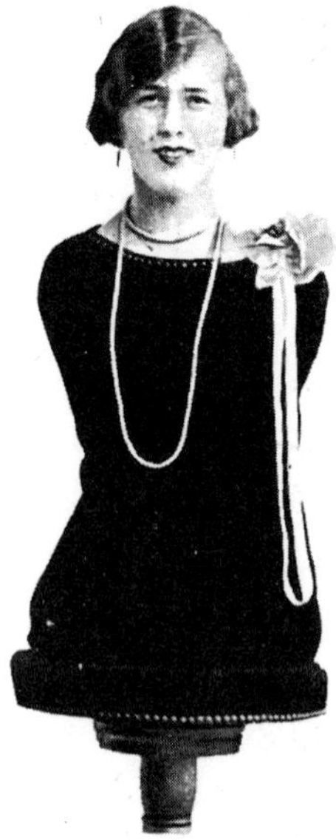

who was born completely deprived of arms but with the rest of the body well formed in the trunk though with some deformity in the feet. Ducornet put this deformity to use, however, since the extra space between the big toe and the second toe enabled him to use his foot like a hand with a thumb. He became so skilful in his chosen calling that he finally painted a picture of Mary Magdalene at the feet of Christ after the Resurrection which was eleven feet high. This picture was bought by the French Government and presented to the corporation of Lille, which was Ducornet's birthplace. ¶ Victorians who had the correct entrée knew well the figure and skeleton of the famous disabled athlete Harvey Leach, kept in the museum of University College Hospital, which had been founded only four years before the Queen's accession. The pelvis was comparatively weak and the thighs hardly recognizable. The right shin and foot were defective, and the left foot, though better shaped, was out of proportion to the trunk. Yet Leach was one of the most remarkable gymnasts of his day, and in spite of the distortion of his lower limbs he displayed a marvellous power and agility in them. As a professional show horseman he was in the first class, 'sitting' his horse sometimes on his buttocks and sometimes standing on his diminutive legs. He walked and even ran quite well, and he had an unusual skill in leaping, partly using his feet and partly his hands. His legs were so short that when he stood he could touch the ground with his fingers, yet he relied on his legs for many of his demonstrations. ¶ Many tricks done with her toes by an armless Hindu woman were described by Curran in 1887 in the London *Medical Press and Circular*. Curran said that this woman, forty years old, worked as a prostitute. The so-called 'Turtle Woman of Demarara' was described in the *Lancet* of 1867, where she was said to have been given the name for two reasons: because her mother was frightened by a turtle during pregnancy, and because as a child she was thought to resemble a turtle. The thighs were only 6 inches long and the feet grew immediately out of them. When this woman was twenty-two she gave birth to a full-grown child free of deformity. She died later of syphilis in the Colonial Hospital. ¶ With regard to supernumerary limbs, probably the most striking is the case of Francesco Lentini, which was discussed earlier. In 1830 Geoffroy Sainte-Hilaire presented to the Académie des Sciences a child with four legs and four feet who was in good clinical health. An instance of three feet on two legs was recorded, one of the legs ending in a double or cloven foot. The reverse effect occurs in the so-called 'Sirens', which are born resembling mermaids. ¶ Parallel to the cloven foot, a double hand has been reported. The subject was a charwoman, and although she leaned on the double hand while scrubbing the floor, and used it to wring out the cloth, she could not summon up as much power in the double hand as in her other, normal, right hand. The absence of fingers in various numbers is a fairly common occurrence, and in one case presented by Köhler in 1893 in the *Berliner klinische Wochenschrift* there was an extraordinary parallel suppression and deformity in both fingers and toes. ¶ Additional fingers and toes are a common occurrence, and few Victorian scientists got excited about the anomaly until they had notched up a sufficiently impressive number. Voight

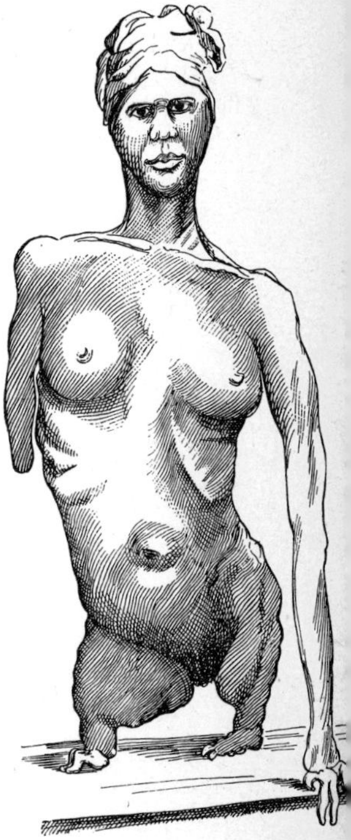

The 'Turtle Woman'.

recorded one instance of thirteen fingers on each hand and twelve toes on each foot. Field research revealed that the incidence of supernumerary digits was often governed by heredity. A family named Foldi discovered in the tribe of the Hyabites living in Arabia were numerous enough to confine their marriages within their own tribe. All in the family had twenty-four digits, and this record was maintained by a simple if barbarous practice: any infant born with the normal number of fingers and toes was sacrificed by slaughter on the grounds that the child must have been adulterously conceived. In one remote and mountainous area of France, in the village of Eycaux, nearly all the inhabitants had a supernumerary digit whether on the hand or the foot. This went on until the coming of better communications opened up the village. The population in part emigrated, and some of those who remained behind married partners who came from outside, and the preponderance of what was called sexdigitism fell away. A family living in Berlin was also recorded whose members had twenty-four digits for many generations, and any woman in it who gave birth to a normal child refused to acknowledge it. The *American Medical Times* located a family in the western territories in which supernumerary digits had lasted through five generations. ¶ The formation of a tail in a human by the prolongation of the coccyx, though occasionally being verified on home ground, was in Victorian times much more widely reported as a fact of life abroad, or in so-called barbarous parts of the country like Cornwall or Ireland. With the growth of exploration this particular quality was annexed for wild races in remote parts. Hubsch of Constantinople reported that both men and women of the Niam-Niam tribe in Central Africa had tails which came either smooth or hairy and could stretch from 2 to 10 inches long. A Wesleyan missionary, George Brown, reported the formal breeding of a tailed race in Kali, off the coast of New Britain, the largest island of the Bismarck Archipelago off the coast of Papua. He said that tail-less children were killed at birth because they would be exposed to public ridicule. The tailed men of Borneo were said to be the result of a hereditary tendency similar to that which produced supernumerary digits. It was confidently asserted that one of the families of princely rulers in Rajputana, lying between the basins of the rivers Indus and Ganges, sported tails and were extremely proud of their ancestral feature. In Europe tails of up to 6 inches in length were reported, but the only one illustrated, in a child, was only 10 centimetres or 4 inches long. All tails were said to be extremely painful, especially when the wearer was riding a horse. ¶ The Paris *Journal de médicine* described a girl of fourteen, otherwise healthy and of good constitution, who had neither external genital organs nor an anus. A plain covering of skin stretched over this area. She ate regularly, but every third day she experienced pain in the region of the navel and much irritation in the intestines. This was followed by severe vomiting of stercoraceous matter. The pains then ceased, and the girl cleansed her mouth with aromatic washes, remaining well until the third day following. Some of the urine was evacuated through the nipples. Fournier narrated that he had been called by three students who had been trying to deliver a woman for five days. He found a woman of apparently good constitution in horrible agony. She said she was twenty-two years old. According to the students she had not had a passage of the bowels for eight days, and Fournier prescribed an enema. The student who tried to give the enema found that the patient had no anus. By putting his finger into the vagina he could discern the floating end of the rectum which was full of faeces. There was an opening in this suspended rectum about the size of an undistended anus. Lavage was undertaken by a cannula introduced through the opening, and a great number of cherry stones agglutinated with faeces followed the water, and labour was soon terminated. The woman afterwards confessed that she was perfectly aware of her deformity, but had been ashamed to disclose it. ¶ Complete absence of the breasts in a body otherwise undoubtedly female has been found very rarely, and when reported was associated with other malfunctions which affected the sex organs. Greenhow in the *Medical-Chirurgical Transactions* of London described a case in which the breasts were absent, but

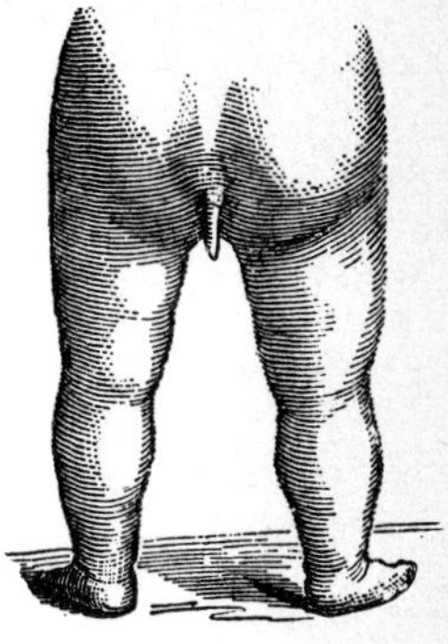

A 4-inch tail on a young child.

there were depressed rudimentary nipples and areolae. The patient had no ovaries, and the uterus was congenitally imperfect. Cases of only one breast existing are more frequent, and on occasion the absence of the breast on one side is associated with the absence of an ovary on the same side. Under-development of the breasts to an anomalous degree is also seen most often in females with associated genital imperfections. Excessive development of the breasts is generally not a congenital condition but results from an acquired disease. But the configuration of the female in certain races does seem to be a permanent hereditary feature, particularly among certain tribes in Central Africa. In women of the Bushman tribe the breasts are naturally very large and pendulous, and mothers normally throw a breast over the shoulder to suckle a child carried on the back. ¶ Polymazia, or the possession of more than the normal pair of breasts, was found by Victorian researchers to be far more common than was generally supposed, and it was said that the existence of extra nipples in males was even more frequent than in females. Gould and Pyle reported in 1896 that they had seen a man with six distinct nipples, 'arranged as regularly as those of a bitch or sow. The two lower were quite small. This man's body was covered with heavy, long hair, making him a very conspicuous object when seen naked during bathing. The hair was absent for a space of nearly an inch about the nipples.' The Cape mulatto woman, portrayed from life in 1881, had six breasts and was said to bear children four or five at a time. ¶ Summing up current research in the *University Medical Magazine* of Philadelphia (May 1896), Hirst wrote: 'Supernumerary breasts and nipples are more common than is generally supposed. Bruce found 60 instances in 3956 persons examined (1.56 per cent.). Leichtenstern places the frequency at one in 500. Both observers declare that men present the anomaly about twice as frequently as women. It is impossible to account for the accessory glands on the theory of reversion, as they occur with no regularity in situation, but may develop at odd places on the body. The most frequent position is on the pectoral surface below the true mammae and somewhat nearer the middle line,

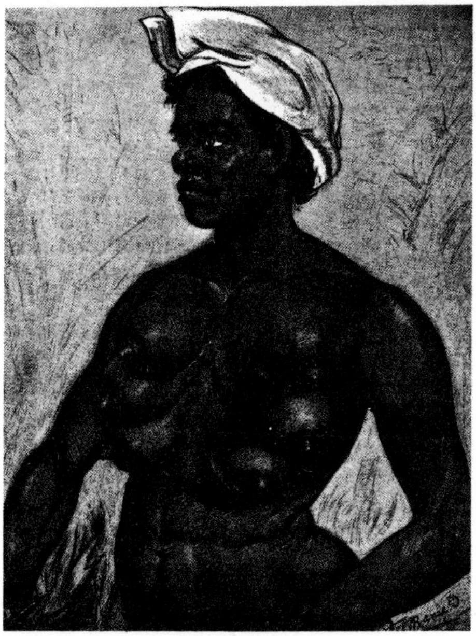

The Cape mulatto woman
with six breasts.

but an accessory gland has been observed on the left shoulder over the prominence of the deltoid [the shoulder-muscle which raises the arm], on the abdominal surface below the costal cartilages [the gristle of the ribs], above the umbilicus [navel], in the axilla [armpit], in the groin, on the dorsal [back] surface, on the labium majus [of the vagina], and on the outer aspect of the left thigh. Ahlfeld explains the presence of mammae on odd parts of the body by the theory that portions of the embryonal material entering into the composition of the mammary gland are carried to and implanted upon any portion of the exterior of the body by means of the amnion [the sac encircling the foetus in the womb].' ¶ The greatest number of supernumerary breasts found by Victorian researchers was ten on one person, reported by Neugebauer in 1886. Other researchers reported some peculiarly placed breasts. 'In the village of Phullendorf in Germany early in [the nineteenth] century there was an old woman who sought alms from place to place, exhibiting to the curious four symmetrical breasts, arranged parallel. She was extremely ugly, and when on all fours, with her breasts pendulous, she resembled a beast.' Hirst, in the article quoted, mentioned a Negress of nineteen years

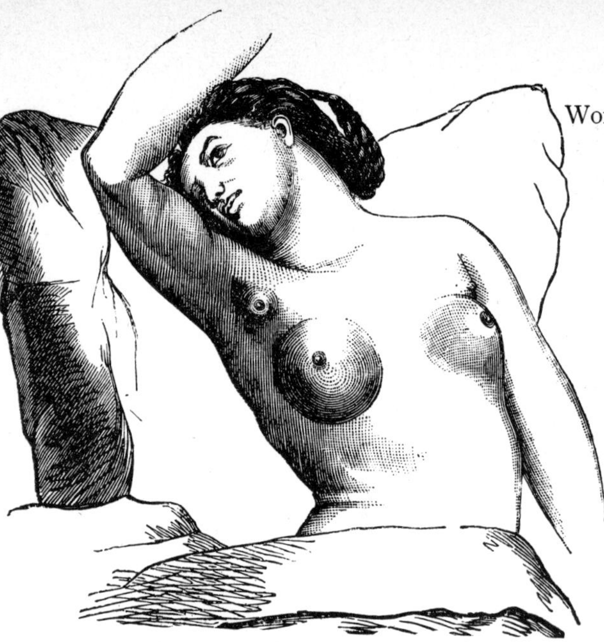

Woman with two axillary breasts.

of age who had nine breasts, all replete with nipples. The two normal glands were very large. Two accessory glands below them were small and did not excrete milk. All the other glands and nipples gave milk in large quantities. There were five nipples on the left and four on the right side. The patient's mother had one accessory breast on the abdomen which secreted milk during the period of lactation. ¶ Some quite diminutive accessory breasts were found to be functional. Charpentier reported that he had received in his clinic a woman with two supplementary mammae in the armpits. They gave milk as the ordinary breasts did. Robert saw a woman who nourished a child from a breast on the thigh which, before pregnancy began, had been taken for an ordinary naevus (mole) but as pregnancy advanced it began to develop and reached the size of a lemon. Some women used a supernumerary breast to suckle more than one child at a time. Jussieu wrote in the *Lancet* of a woman who had three breasts, one of which was situated in the groin and with which she occasionally suckled; her mother had three breasts, but they were all situated on the chest. Martin in the *Archive für klinische Chirurgie* of 1893 printed a clear illustration of a woman with one supernumerary breast below the natural organ. ¶ Supernumerary nipples alone were also reported, as many as five having been

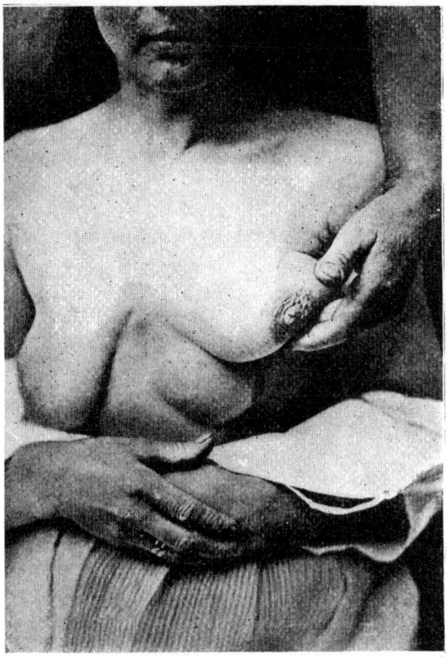

A supernumerary breast.

found on the same breast. In one case reported by Neugebauer there were eight accessory nipples. Hollerus wrote of a woman he had seen who had two nipples on the same breast which gave milk with the same regularity and the same abundance as the other, single nipple. ¶ Duplication of the hymen began to be mentioned with some frequency after Cornil had made the first report of this condition in 1876. Deficiency in the vulva may be caused by the persistence of a thick hymen but is more often due to congenital occlusion (closure of the orifice at birth) or to complete absence of the vagina, which was occasionally reported. The *Lancet* declared in an issue of 1872 that Vicq d'Azir had seen two females who, not having a vagina, copulated all through life by the urethra. This practice was also reported of a New York prostitute by Ferguson in 1883. In the *Medical Times and Gazette* of London (1852), Brodhurst reported an instance where both vagina and uterus were absent in a girl of sixteen who at four years of age had shown signs of approaching puberty. At this early age the mons veneris was covered with hair, and at ten the clitoris was 3 inches long and 2 inches in circumference. The

The Hottentot labial 'apron' spread out to the sides.

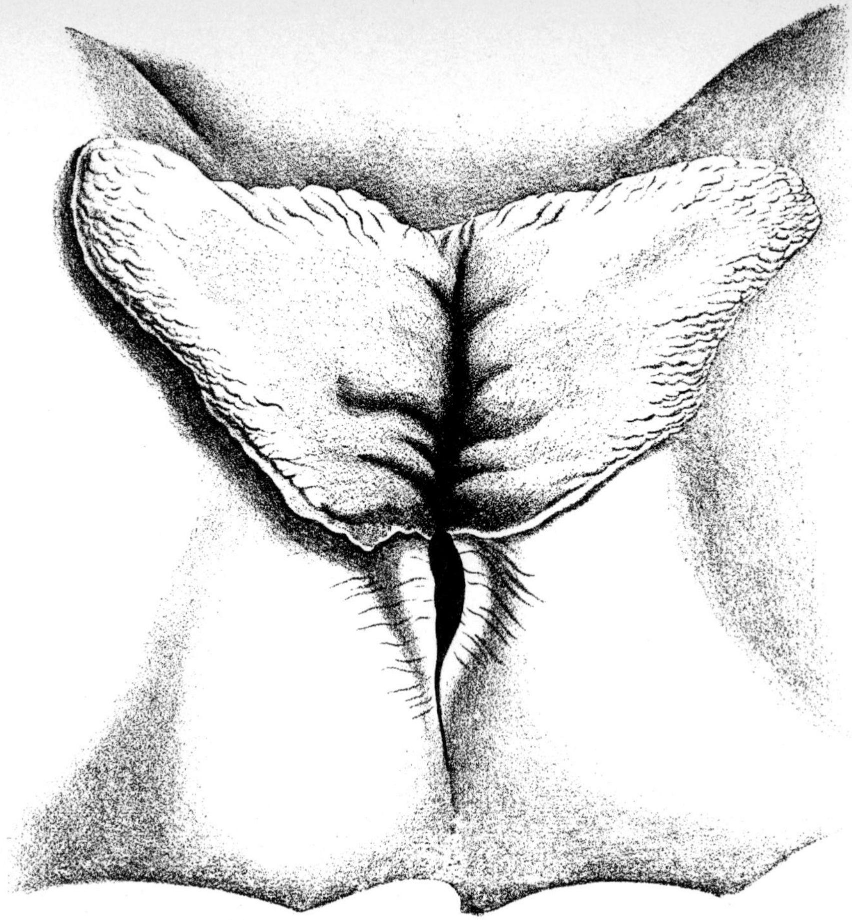

breasts were well developed. The lips of the vulva descended and expanded into folds resembling a scrotum. ¶ Duplication of the vagina was frequently observed by Victorian physicians, and occasionally anomalous openings of the vagina into other parts. Absence of the labia majora was found more often than absence of the labia minora. Enlargement of the labia minora was found to be associated with exaggerated growth of the clitoris. Peculiarities of the two sets of lips in the vulva were particularly noticed by medical men working in Africa, where there was a long history of manipulation of these parts. But it was stated that in China 'the peculiar conditions under which the Chinese women are obliged to live, particularly their mode of sitting, has the effect of causing unusual development of the mons veneris and the labia majora.' 'On the other hand,' a reliable account went on, 'some of the lower African races have been distinguished by the deficiency in development of the labia majora, mons veneris, and genital hair. In this respect they present an approximation to the genitals of the anthropoid apes, among whom the orang-outang alone shows any tendency to formation of the labia majora. ¶ 'The labial appendages of the Hottentot female have been celebrated for many years. Blumenbach and others of the earlier travelers found that the apron-like appearance of the genitals of the Hottentot women was due to abnormal hypertrophy [exaggerated growth] of the labia and nymphae [labia minora]. According to John Knott, the French traveler, Le Vaillant, said that the more coquettish among the Hottentot girls are excited by extreme vanity to practise artificial elongation of the nympha and labia. They are said to pull and rub these parts, and even to stretch them by hanging weights to them. Some of them are said to spend several hours a day at this process, which is considered one of the important parts of the toilet of the Hottentot belle, this malformation being an attraction for the male members of the race. Merensky says that in Basutoland the elder women begin to practise labial manipulation on their female children shortly after infancy, and Adams* has found this custom to prevail in Dahomey; he says that the King's seraglio includes 3000 members, the elect of his female subjects, all of whom have labia up to the standard of recognized length. Cameron found an analogous practice among the women of the shores of Lake Tanganyika. The females of this nation manipulated the skin of the lower part of the abdomens of the female children from infancy, and at puberty these women exhibit a cutaneous curtain [that is, of skin] over the genitals which reaches half-way down the thighs. ¶ 'A corresponding development of the preputian clitorides, attaining the length of 18 mm. or even more, has been observed among the females of Bechuanaland. The greatest elongation measured by Barrow was five inches, but it is quite probable that it was not possible for him to examine the longest, as the females so gifted generally

* This account is confirmed in *Waitz' Introd. Anthropol.* I, 106: 'Adams reports that in Dahomey the nymphae are artificially elongated.' See *Oxford English Dictionary*, ref: Nympha. The translation of Waitz' work was published in 1863.

occupied very high social positions.' ¶ Abnormal enlargement of the clitoris without manipulation was occasionally recorded, the longest known being set down in the *Dictionnaire des sciences médicales* as 'thirty centimetres [12 inches] long and resembling the neck of a goose'. Enlargement of the clitoris to a magnitude which prevented coitus constituted a legitimate cause for divorce in nineteenth-century France. ¶ Rudimentary development of the penis was generally reported as associated with cryptorchidism (failure of one or both of the testicles to descend into the scrotum) or some other abnormality of the male sexual organs. Occasionally an undeveloped penis was restored to normal proportions by normal practice. Wilson, a London doctor who specialized in these matters in the 1850s and 1860s, was once consulted by a gentleman of twenty-six who, as a later work put it, was doubtful about 'his ability to perform the marital function. In size his penis and testicles hardly exceeded those of a boy of eight. He had never felt desire for sexual intercourse until he became acquainted with his intended wife, since when he had erections and nocturnal emissions. The patient married and became the father of a family; those parts which at twenty-six were so much smaller than usual had increased at twenty-eight to normal adult size.' ¶ Cases were noted where the penis was twisted, sometimes permanently by arthritis, once temporarily by freezing, but most often by hypospadias, the malformation of the urethra's lower wall so that the urethra opens on the under-surface of the penis. In *Transactions of the Medical Society of the State of New York*, Gray mentioned a pathetic case of a man suffering from this disability, later summed up as follows: 'When he determined to get married, fully appreciating his physical defect, he resolved to imitate nature, and being of a very ingenious turn of mind, he busied himself with the construction of an artificial penis. While so engaged he had seized every opportunity to study the conformation of this organ, and finally prepared a body formed of cotton, six inches in length, and shaped like a penis, minus a prepuce. He sheathed it in pig's gut and gave it a slight vermilion hue. To the touch it felt elastic, and its shape was maintained by a piece of gutta-percha tubing, around which the cotton was firmly wound. It was fastened to the waistband by means of straps, a central and an upper one being so arranged that the penis could be thrown into an erect position and so maintained. He had constructed a flesh-coloured covering which completely concealed the straps. With this artificial member he was enabled to deceive his wife for fifteen months, and was only discovered when she undressed him in a state of intoxication. To further the deception he had told his wife immediately after their marriage that it was quite indecent for a husband to undress in the presence of his wife, and therefore she had always retired first and turned out the light. Partly from fear that his virile power would be questioned and partly from ignorance, the duration of actual coitus would approach an hour. When the discovery was made, his wife hid the instrument with which he had perpetrated a most successful fraud upon her, and the patient subsequently attempted coitus by contact, with unsuccessful results, although both parties had incomplete orgasms. Shortly afterward evidences of mental derangement appeared and the man became the subject of exalted delusions. His wife, at the time of report, had filed application for divorce.' ¶ Entire absence of the male sexual apparatus is extremely rare, but two cases were cited from Victorian times. Complete absence of the testicles was reported as being almost as rare, though it was difficult to distinguish cases of congenital absence from others involving arrested development or simple atrophy. Men with only one testicle, known as monorchids, were sometimes found to have the solitary testicle divided in the middle by a deep fissure, the two lobes being each provided with a spermatic cord on the same side as the lobe. The existence of polyorchids, persons with more than two testicles, was for long not credited, but in his *chef d'œuvre* published in 1833, which he entitled *Observations on Testicles*, a Scottish expert on the subject, Dr Russell of Edinburgh, mentioned four, five, and even six testicles in one individual, though not every case he mentioned was verified by dissection. In one that was verified, however, he discovered six testicles in a scrotum, four of the usual size and two smaller than ordinary. Russell mentioned a monk who was endowed with three testicles, and was so salacious that he was unable to keep his vows of chastity. The amorous propensities and generative faculties of polyorchids were always supposed in Victorian times to be greater than ordinary, and Russell reported another case of a triorchid who was prescribed a concubine as a reasonable allowance to a man thus endowed. Following Russell's *magnum opus* doctors appear to have taken the possibility of polyorchidism more seriously, and in 1865 the *Lancet* reported that three cases of triorchidism had been found in the British army. Such cases were generally discovered during post-mortem examinations after death in battle, but if this condition was discovered by palpation (handling) in the ordinary medical examination of a British soldier, no extreme action seems to have been taken. In the Russian army, however, the soldier was discharged as a man subject to abnormal temptation who might consequently lead his comrades astray. The *London Medical Record* in 1884 quoted a report by the Russian Dr Bulatoff mentioning a soldier who had a third testicle, the diagnosis being confirmed by several of Bulatoff's colleagues. 'They recommended dismissal of the man from the service, as the third testicle, usually resting in some portion of the inguinal canal, caused extra exposure to traumatic influence.' ¶ It is fair to say of the last case quoted that a testicle positioned in the inguinal canal (in the groin, in the passage usually occupied only by the spermatic cord) would possibly cause unexpected pain at an awkward moment in battle or during any other activity if the reason it could not descend from the inguinal canal was that the scrotum was already fully occupied. But in an appreciable proportion of cryptorchids, that is, men whose testicles are still in the abdominal cavity, these testicles are found in the inguinal canal. Of 89 cases of cryptorchidism collated by Dr Johnson in the *Transactions of the Medical and Chirurgical Faculty of Maryland* in 1884 – and all these reports were made from post-mortems – both testicles were found in the inguinal canal in 18 cases, and in 8 other cases one testicle was found in this position, the other not appearing at all. Of 16 cases in which the semen was examined microscopically during life, there were 3 in which spermatozoa were found. But 10 of the total subjects had had children. ¶ There were a number of cases where the testicle was more gravely displaced, in the perineum, in the abdomen, or lying against the pubic bone. After Russell's remarkable work on the subject, British military and naval physicians paid particular attention to the testicles of serving men, the more so when it was shown that apparent cryptorchidism could be used as a means of malingering or even dodging military service altogether. The classic case, cited by Russell, concerned an English merchant seaman whose ship, according to the custom of the time, had been boarded by a recruiting party from H.M.S. *Druid* off the coast of Africa, and the boarding-party had pressed the seaman into service with the Royal Navy. The man declared that he was unfit to serve. 'He said he had been examined by dozens of ship-surgeons, but was invariably rejected on account of rupture in both groins. The scrotum was found to be an empty bag, and close examination showed that the testicles occupied the seats of the supposed rupture. As soon as the discovery was made the man became unnerved and agitated, and on re-examining the parts the testicles were found in the scrotum. When he found that there was no chance for escape he acknowledged that he was an impostor and gave an exhibition in which, with incredible facility, he pulled both testes up from the bottom of the scrotum to the external abdominal ring. At the word of command he could pull up one testicle, then another, and let them drop simultaneously; he performed other like feats so rapidly that the movements could not be distinguished.' ¶ Other curiosities mentioned by Russell included 'a man whose testicle was elevated every time the east wind blew, which caused him a sense of languor and relaxation', and 'a man whose testicles ascended into the inguinal canal every time he was in the company of women'.

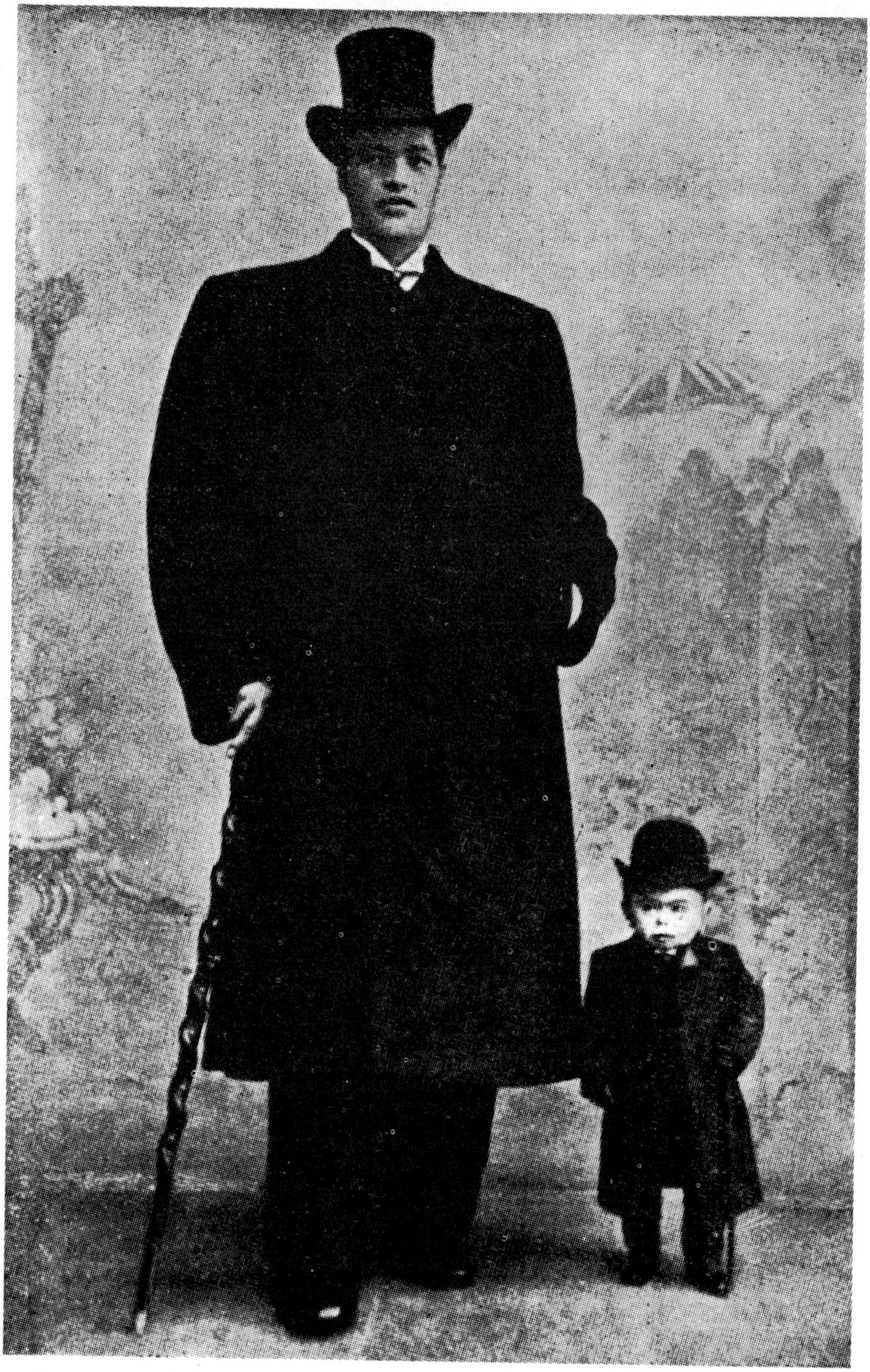

Victorian contrasts – giant and dwarf.

CHAPTER FOUR

GIANTS, DWARFS, FAT LADIES AND LIVING SKELETONS

GIANTS are the real stuff of Barnum & Bailey for, unless you are looking face-to-face (or face-to-navel) at a giant in person, there is no way to convey his great size except by picturing him alongside ordinary people – or preferably as a cloud-capped tower poised menacingly over a dwarf. If the two can be persuaded to marry, so much the better. The Victorians had a music hall joke concerning a very tall guardsman who fell in love with a very short lady and asked advice about the prospects of such a union, enquiring, 'Do you think we shall get on?' The answer given was, 'You'll get on all right, but you'll have no one to talk to.' The Parisians had a more untranslatable joke about the marriage of a giant on the fourth of July, 1897. ¶ Gigantism has always been in the area of myth, and in the nineteenth century the myths were encouraged by false statistics put out by the showmen who exhibited giants. Even today, circus giants and dwarfs are generally signatories to a contract which forbids them to be measured, so that exaggerated claims can be made for them. Authentic measuring of extreme height or depth in humans began only a few years before Victoria's time, and the records were collated by Charles Dana in 1895. According to Dana, the number of giants figuring as public characters since 1700 was not more than a hundred, and of these about twenty were advertised as being 8 feet tall. Since it is known that promotional advertising falsely exaggerated the stature of most of these, who were not reliably measured by any medical man in any case, very few can in reality have exceeded 8 feet. Of those giants known to the Victorians who had been accurately and scientifically measured, Winckelmeyer of Germany is known to have been 8 feet 6 inches tall. Ranke measured Marianne Wehde, another German, and found that she measured 8 feet 4¼ inches when only sixteen years old – a truly extraordinary height for a woman. Topinard measured the tallest man in the Austrian army and recorded his height as 8 feet 4½ inches. But undoubtedly the tallest with impeccable references known to the Victorians was Machnov, 'the Russian Giant', who attained a height of 9 feet 4¼ inches. When he died there succeeded to the title a shorter monster, Hugo, who went on show at the Paris Exhibition and whose statistics bring to life the whole business, and problems, of walking tall. ¶ Hugo was born in the Alpes-Maritimes. At twenty-two years of age he was 7 feet 6 inches tall and weighed 443 lb., or 31 stone 9 lb. By stretching his arm up he reached a point well over 10 feet high. With his arms extended he could reach points over 8 feet apart. He measured 75 inches round the chest. His bed was 10 feet long and 5 feet wide. The height of his father was 5 feet 4½ inches, of his mother 5 feet 6 inches – and his brother was rejected for service in the army because of his short stature. At birth Hugo weighed 15 lb. At the age of six he was over 4 feet tall, at fifteen he was 6 feet 6 inches, and at twenty-two he was still growing by almost an inch a year. ¶ Generally with giants the great stature is due to excessive growth of the thighs and legs, the size of the head and the trunk being nearly the same as in normal persons of comparable age. On the other hand, in a natural

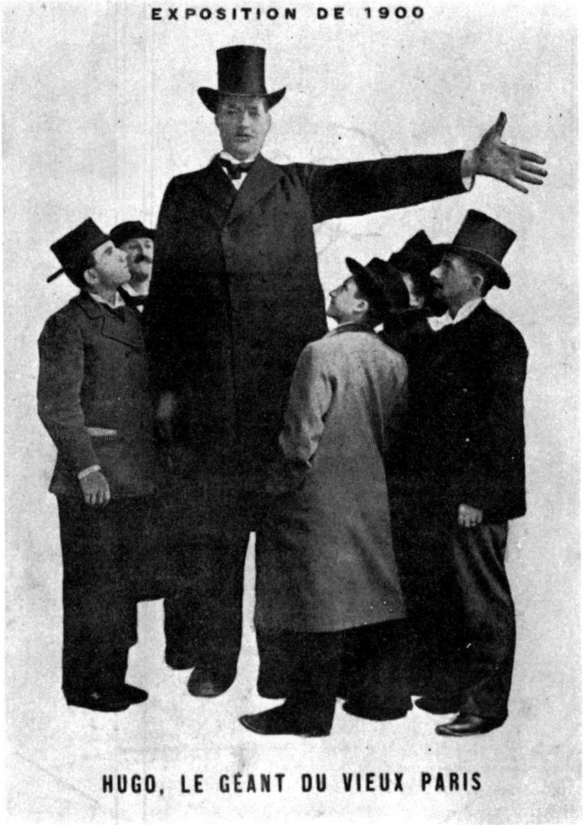

Hugo, 7 feet 6 inches tall, at the Paris Exhibition in 1900.

dwarf, the proportions are fairly uniform, the head however being always larger in proportion to the body, as is normally the case with children. The proportions of General Tom Thumb, who has been mentioned previously, were those of an ordinary child aged between thirteen and fifteen months. Towards the end of the nineteenth century an association was recognized between gigantism and acromegaly, a disease marked by enlargement of the face, hands, and feet caused by a pathological condition of the pituitary gland. But in giants there generally seemed to be an acquired uniform enlargement of all the lower bones of the body. In 1895 Brissaud and Meige described in the *Journal de médicine et de chirurgie praticale* the case of a male aged forty-seven who had shown no signs of unusual development before the age of sixteen. He then began to grow larger, until at twenty-one he measured 7 feet 2 inches in height and weighed about 340 lb. He remained well and very strong until the age of thirty-seven, when he overlifted, and following this he developed an extreme deformity of the spine and trunk, the latter 'telescoping into itself' until the nipples were on a level with the anterior superior spines of the ilium (that is, roughly level with the hip bone). For two years he suffered with debility, fatigue, bronchitis, night-sweats, headache, and great thirst. Mentally he was dull. The bones of his face and the extremities showed the hypertrophies (exaggerated growth) characteristic of acromegaly, the soft parts not being involved. The circumference of the trunk at the nipples was 62 inches, and over the most prominent part of the kyphosis (humped back) and pigeon breast it was 74 inches. Gould and Pyle in 1896 stressed the striking resemblance of the disproportionate growth of a boy in adolescence to the classic description of acromegaly: that the disease manifests itself in the bones of the extremities and in the extremities of the bones. And they hazarded the proposition: 'Acromegaly is gigantism of the adult; gigantism is acromegaly of adolescence.'

¶ There is no doubt of the special place occupied by giants in history, although the actual records of their measurement may justifiably be scrutinized with extreme suspicion. Very often they were sought for privileged positions, or at least such prominent positions (not necessarily overpaid) as being sentries outside a royal palace or members of a royal bodyguard. Harrison Ainsworth, the Victorian writer of historical fiction, said that the Tower of London was guarded in 1553 by three brothers claiming direct descent from Henry VIII, whose names were Og, Gog, and Magog and who were all over 8 feet in height. The names Gog and Magog occur variously in the Bible, and in the last reference, in the Book of Revelation, they are considered to be a comprehensive term for the power of evil. But in England Gogmagog was the name of one traditional giant until it was split into two to refer to British giants who fought against the Trojan invaders of Britain under Brutus, the mythical conqueror who was supposed to have given his name to Britain. Whether Ainsworth's fanciful giants could justify any blood relationship with King Henry VIII is an even more doubtful matter. 'Claiming direct descent', they could just about have been his grandsons if he had sired their parent by 1510, when he was nineteen. If they were his sons, history has recorded no woman to whom Henry was constant enough, or whom he was, apparently, potent enough, to have impregnated on three separate occasions, which could only have been between the years 1522, when he decided to divorce Catherine of Aragon, and 1533, when he married Anne Boleyn. ¶ Among other bodyguards to kings and noblemen were the famous Company of Giants in the Foot Guards of Frederick the Great of Prussia. The yeomen of the guard of one of the Dukes of Hanover, Christopher Munster, were said to be 8 feet 6 inches tall. 'Big Sam', the porter at Carlton House when it was the home of the Prince Regent, later King George IV, was 8 feet tall. Queen Elizabeth I's porter, whose painted portrait can be seen at Hampton Court, was 7 feet 6 inches. Walter Parson, porter to Elizabeth's successor, James I, was about the same height. William Evans, who filled the same position for King Charles I, was reputed to be nearly 8 feet tall and he certainly carried a dwarf in his pocket, like a lap-dog. In any exchange of witticisms between the pair, however, it is likely that Evans came off the worst. During his lifetime a courtier set out to amuse the Empress of Austria by summoning a congress of all giants and dwarfs in the Empire. The giants eventually lodged a complaint to the court that the dwarfs teased them so unmercifully that they were making their lives thoroughly miserable. ¶ In the year of Victoria's accession a young man went on show advertised as being 'formerly in the service of the King of the Netherlands' (he was probably discharged when the Netherlands were broken up and Victoria's uncle, Leopold, became King of the Belgians). He was 8 feet 10 inches tall and weighed 401 lb. At this time medical researchers were becoming so interested in specimens of extreme growth that they tended to hunt them down like body-snatchers, but tactlessly made their mission known long before the deaths of their intended subjects, so that the sensitive giants lived in morbid fear of dissection. This was the nightmare of the celebrated 'Irish Giant' O'Brien, who was reputed to be 8 feet 4 inches tall. O'Brien became aware that his skeleton had long been sought by John Hunter, the famous Scottish anatomist and the most brilliant pioneer surgeon in medical history. Hunter had made a vow that he would have the skeleton of 'the Irish Giant', and O'Brien made a counter-vow that he would not, being somewhat averse to being boiled in the distinguished scientist's kettle. (The kettle in which bodies were boiled before stripping was not the spouted teatime variety, but a huge cauldron.) The giant was tormented all his life by repeated reminders of Hunter's oath to have him and by the spies which the surgeon constantly set to report on his movements. O'Brien, like many giants, developed a sickly disposition and deteriorated early in his life. When he was on his deathbed he paid some fishermen to take his body after his death and sink it in the middle of the Irish Channel with heavy weights attached. But Hunter's spies reported this development to their master. Hunter then over-bribed the fishermen and got possession of the body. It was calculated that it cost Hunter over five hundred pounds in good eighteenth-century money to secure the skeleton of 'the Irish Giant'. The kettle in which the body was boiled was preserved in the museum of the Royal College of Surgeons and exhibited at a meeting of the British Medical Association in 1895. The skeleton became one of the features of the museum, actually measuring 92¾ inches in height, and was displayed mounted alongside the skeleton of Carolina Crachami, a Sicilian dwarf, exhibited in London during her lifetime as 'the Italian Princess', who died at the age of nine. Most of the 13,000 specimens bequeathed by Hunter to the Royal College of Surgeons were destroyed in an air raid in 1941. Curiously, the original statues of Gog and Magog in the Guildhall, London, were destroyed in the Great Fire of 1666. Replicas were made in 1708 and destroyed in the historic air raid which nearly blotted out St Paul's Cathedral on 29 December 1940. New figures of the giants were made for the Festival of Britain in 1951. ¶ Among the giants familiar to the Victorians was Chang Yu Sing, 'the

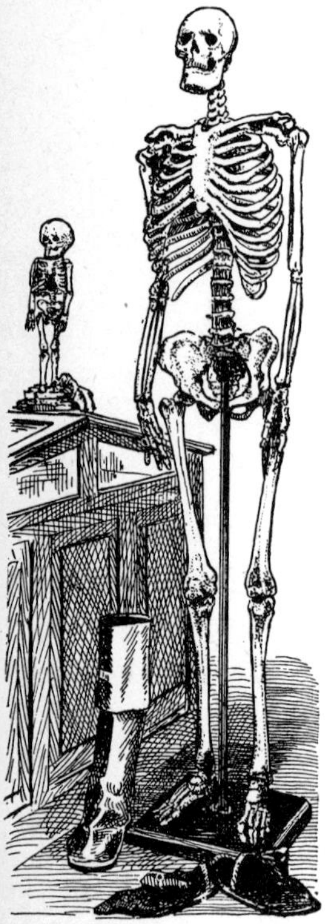

Skeleton of the Irish giant, O'Brien.

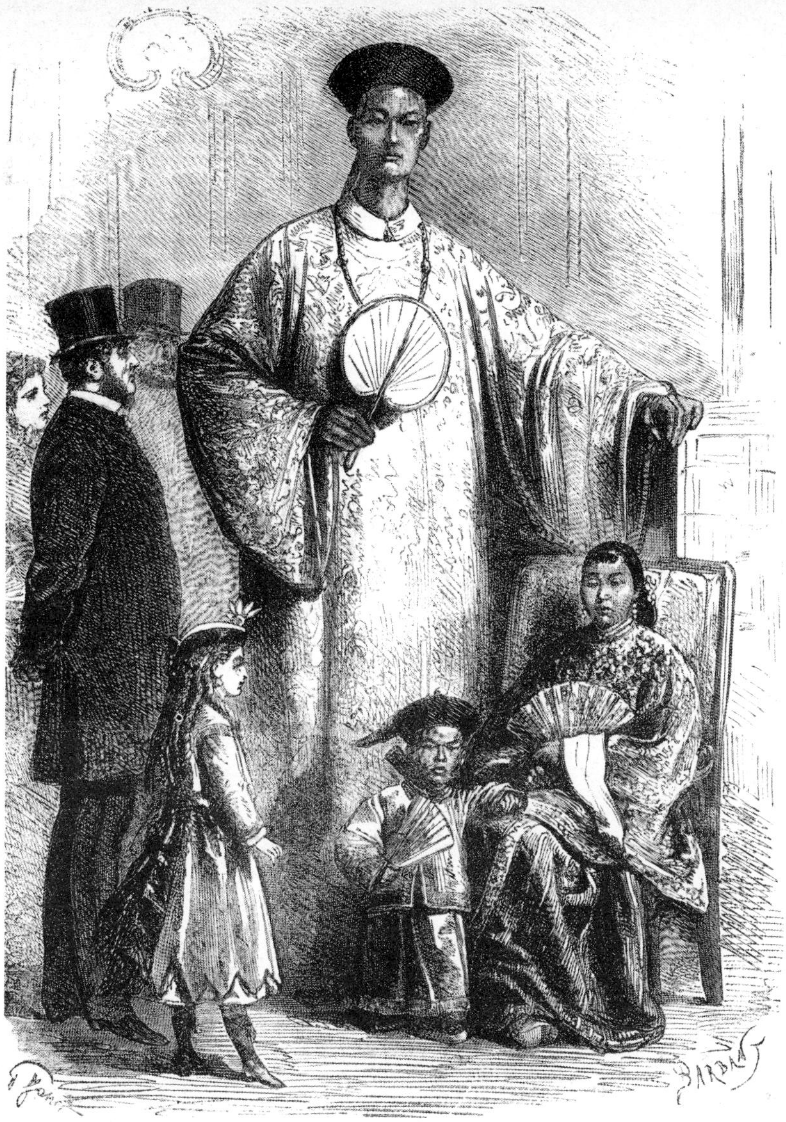

Chang Yu Sing, 'the Chinese giant', who approached 8 feet in height.

Chinese Giant', who approached 8 feet in height. He had a passion for jewels, gold and pearls, and preferred to be clothed in red velvet, embroidered silk, and panther-skin. He was known as the aristocrat of giants. ¶ Among well-known women giants was Leah the Giantess, who was 7 feet 2 inches tall at the age of nineteen, and Miss Marian, 'Queen of the Amazons', who measured half an inch over 8 feet when she was eighteen. In 1882 a special show was written around her for her appearance at the Alhambra in London, and the entertainment, entitled *Babil and Bijou,* was a great success. Miss Marian came on stage wearing a striking costume covered with pearls and apparently precious stones, and a Babylonian helmet hoisted her height by another ten inches. ¶ 'The Nova Scotia Giantess', Anna H. Swann, was 7 feet 5½ inches in height, though the showmen for whom she worked claimed that she was 8 feet 1 inch. While she was on tour in England she met a man who was slightly her inferior, Captain Martin Van Buren Bates, standing 7 feet 2½ inches. Captain Bates, born in Kentucky in 1845, enlisted in the Southern army during the American Civil War in 1861, and although only sixteen years old he was accepted because of his size. At the end of the war Captain Bates had attained his full height and weighed 450 lb., not through excess fat, for he had a well-proportioned body. As soon as the two giants met in London they fell in love, and they were married at St Martin in the Fields in the summer of 1871. After this they went on tour together, and with a combined height of 14 feet 8 inches were beyond reasonable doubt the tallest married couple known to mankind. Anna died seventeen years later, but the captain survived until his seventy-fourth year, dying in 1919. The captain's father was 5 feet 10 inches tall, and his mother 5 feet 3 inches. Anna's father was 6 feet tall and her mother 5 feet 2 inches. ¶ In the *Medical Record* of New York (22 March 1879), Beach gives an invaluable account of the birth of Captain Bates' child to Anna. Labour was slow, but she was successfully delivered of a healthy child which was 30 inches long (against an average of 18 to 20 inches) and 23¾ lb. in weight (some three times heavier than the average). The afterbirth weighed 10 lb. and the quantity of amniotic fluid was 9 quarts. The weight of 23¾ lb. was in Victorian days the heaviest on record for any authenticated single birth. A report in Haller's *Bibliotheca Chirurgica* of 1774, quoting Mittehauser, had spoken of a newborn child weighing 24 lb., but there were no details and only slight authentication of the actual figure. But in the year 1884 the *Lancet* (vol. ii, p. 1029) printed a report by Warren that he had delivered a woman in Derbyshire of male twins, one weighing 17 lb. 8 oz., and the other 18 lb. The placenta weighed 4 lb., and there was an ordinary pailful of liquid amnii. The parents were of normal stature. Both the twins were muscular and well-formed and had an excellent chance of surviving. ¶ At the reverse extreme, boy and girl twins were born to Mrs J. B. McCrum of Kalamazoo, Michigan, in 1874 weighing 1 lb. 8 oz. and 1 lb. 12 oz., and each could be held in the palm of a nurse's hand. Premature female twins weighing 22½ and 24 oz. were born in 1858 in England and followed well into adult life, the *British Medical Journal* reporting in 1884 that the larger twin had married and borne two children. At birth a wedding ring could easily be passed over the hand, forearm, and arm of her smaller sister. ¶ The death of a giant, particularly in a high building, sometimes posed problems. When William Campbell, a Scot approaching 7 feet, died in Newcastle in 1878, the window and wall of the room in which he expired had to be taken out, frame and brickwork down to the floor, so that the coffin could be lowered by block and tackle three storeys to the ground. Robert Wadlow, a post-Victorian giant who died in St Louis, Missouri, in 1940 at the age of twenty-two and measuring 8 feet 11.1 inches, was buried in Oakwood, Illinois, in a coffin 10 feet 9 inches long, 32 inches wide, and 30 inches deep. He weighed 439 lb. (31 stone 5 lb.) at the time of his death, but in his prime had turned the scales at nearly four stone heavier, 491 lb. ¶ Gigantism is caused by over-activity of the anterior lobe of the pituitary gland. If the excessive secretion of the growth hormone of the pituitary commences during the normal period of growth a giant is produced. If the hypersecretion occurs after adolescence there is no general increase in stature but an enlargement of the bones of the face, hands, and feet, which has already been noted as acromegaly, because of the stimulating effect of the hormone upon growth. With this condition there may be an over-growth of hair on the chest and the appearance of hair on the face of women, often coupled with signs of over-stimulation of the sex functions as an indication of the over-production of other hormones of the anterior lobe of the pituitary – the gonadotrophic hormones and others. When there is *deficiency* of the anterior lobe secretion in childhood, the result is dwarfism. ¶ There are two main types of pituitary dwarf. In the first, the diminutive body is of normal proportions, but the normality is the normality of development of the *child* – that is, the head remains large by comparison with the rest of the body, following the proportions of an infant. These subjects may or may not show failure of sexual development. They are usually intelligent, of attractive appearance, not so much creatures who are deformed as humans who have been scaled down. They are what we call midgets. In the second type of pituitary dwarf obesity and arrested sexual development are usually apparent. The children are often mentally subnormal, frequently lethargic to the point of going to sleep 'all over the place', and combine this languor with a voracious appetite. When Dickens portrayed the

Examples of pituitary dwarfs.

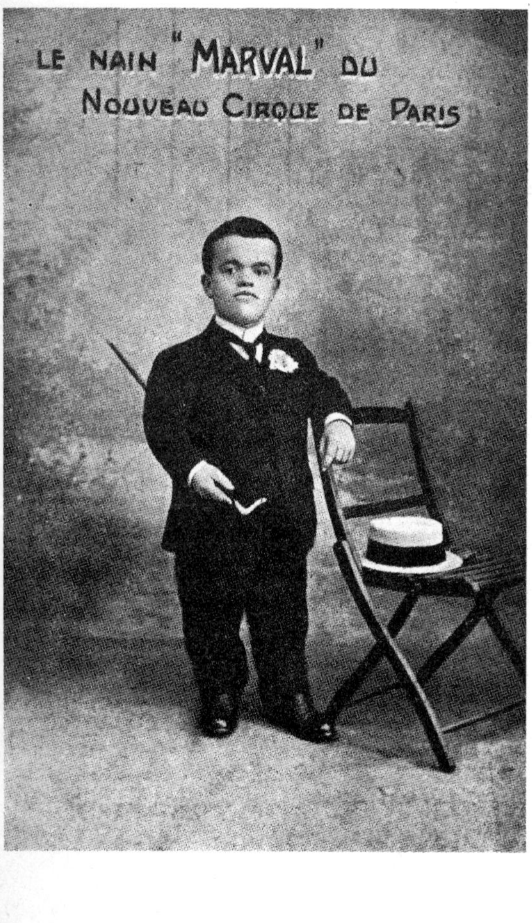

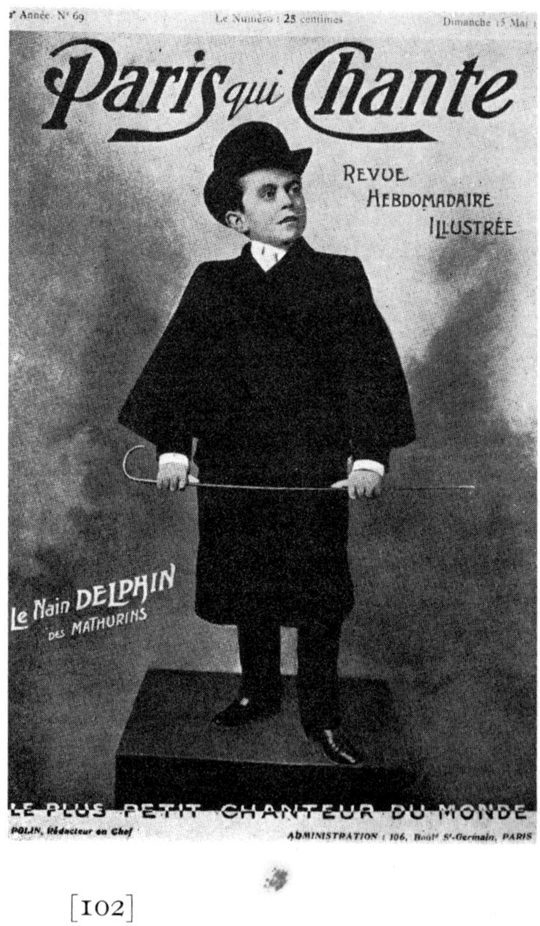

Fat Boy in *The Pickwick Papers* he clearly had a model of this type in his mind. ¶ When this hormone deficiency occurs in adolescents or adults, dwarfing does not present itself. But often there is extreme obesity. The sex functions are suppressed. In the male the fat, besides being excessive, has a feminine distribution, over the hips, thighs, and chest. Hair is scarce or absent on the face, though plentiful on the head, and there is a tendency towards effeminacy in disposition. ¶ Heredity does not seem to play an important part in dwarfism. But there is a distinction between those individuals who through glandular deficiency fall noticeably short of the stature of their parents, and those people such as pygmies, whose stature is normal for their race. The Victorians, bursting with the energy of exploration, seemed to discover pygmies all over the world. The explorer Dr Schweinfurth came back from Africa declaring that everything said on the subject by Homer, Herodotus, and Aristotle was perfectly true, and there was a race of pygmies near the source of the Nile. He said they lived south of the Niam-Niam country, and their stature varied between 4 feet and 4 feet 10 inches in height. He declared that the incredible cunning and agility of these people, called the Akkas, were rare compensations for their small stature. In 1860, Paul DuChaillu returned from another part of Africa, the Ashango country, with tales of another race of pygmies, called the Obongos, who averaged a little over 4 feet in height. Battel went scouting in this region, just south of the Equator, and discovered a further pygmy people, next door to the Obongos, called the Dongos. Kolle took up the challenge and reported the existence of the Kenkobs, who, he said, were only between 3 and 4 feet tall, and in addition there were the Reebas, who could sink as low as 3 feet but sometimes reached 5 feet. The Portuguese claimed that in their own African territory there were dwarf peoples whom they had not bothered to mention before, known as the Bakka-Bakka and the Yogas. Someone reported a Nubian tribe of midgets called the Sukus. India throbbed with stories – more accurately classified as legends – about dwarf tribes descended from the monkey-god Hoonuman.

Examples of two Cotta tribesmen, each standing 3 feet 6 inches high.

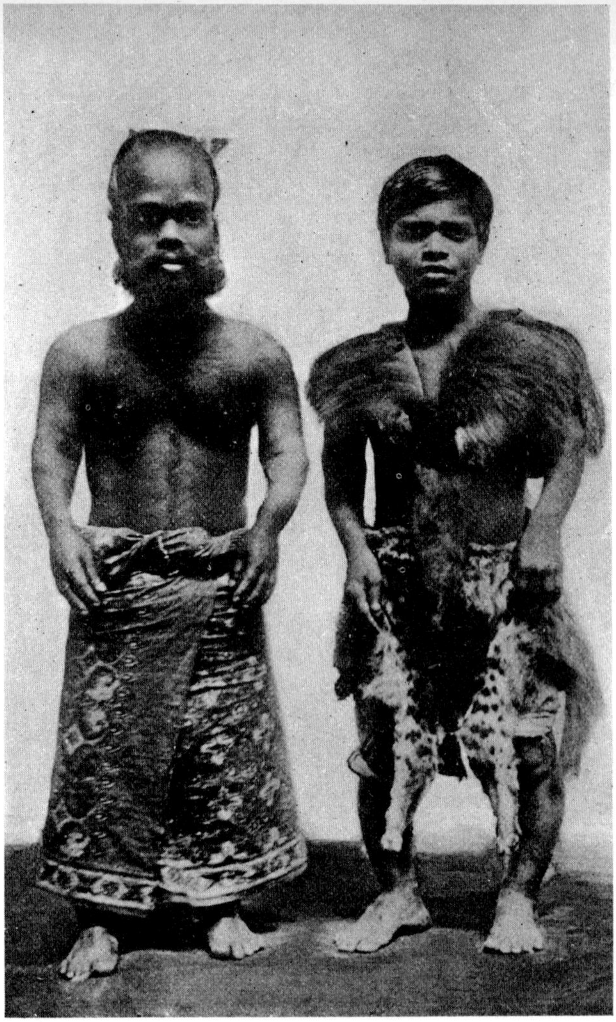

And, in an effort to show that pygmies were not necessarily a tropical people, some Arctic explorers recorded an Eskimo tribe of very small stature whom they had come across. ¶ The search spread to Central America, where 'the Aztec Children', already mentioned and illustrated, were found and brought back to a life of show business in the United States. An expedition of anthropologists set out to comb a hitherto unexplored region near the Isthmus of Tehuantepec in Central America, which had previously been alluded to by Humboldt as the home of a race of pygmies. Professor Starr of Chicago eventually returned to report that he had found many colonies of undersized people but hardly any pygmies. Nevertheless, a rival expedition brought back two Cotta tribesmen, dwarfs standing 3 feet 6 inches high. ¶ An Italian explorer, Miani, set off for the Akka country reported by Schweinfurth near the source of the Nile. He did not reach it, but arrived at the court of King Munza of Monbuttu, where he happened to see two Akka dwarfs who were being kept by the king as curiosities. Miani made a deal with the king and began his journey home with the dwarfs. But the party were ambushed on the way back, and only one of the original expedition survived – a Sudanese sergeant, who had been put in charge of the dwarfs since he had some faint understanding of their language. In his escape he took the dwarfs with him and brought them triumphantly to Rome. They were presented to the King of Italy and took up residence at their new court. They were then about ten and fifteen years old, and their dialect was different from any other African tongue, though the sergeant, with his initial understanding, gradually formed a lingua franca which they could use. When the King of Italy grew tired of them the dwarfs were put in the care of the Royal Geographical Society of Italy. In 1874 the *Lancet* sent a commission to examine and report on them. They were then about 3 feet 9 inches and 3 feet 3 inches tall respectively. As for their temperament, 'they were intelligent in their manner, but resented being lionized too much, and were prone to scratch ladies who attempted to kiss them'. ¶ The Victorians were aware that in ancient times the old emperors, and others who shared their partiality for a few dwarfs around the palace, had attempted the production of artificial dwarfs, generally by starving promising youngsters who were of a sufficiently small stature when they were born. Most of the dwarfs bred in this fashion died from rickets, but those who survived were highly prized by the Roman emperors for their grotesque appearance. In the Middle Ages, when those in the know thought they could do almost anything with the right ointment – even fly on a broomstick by rubbing the correct lotion into the thighs – they concocted a dwarfing mixture from the fat of bats, moles, dormice, and other diminutive animals. But the Victorian showmen, pragmatic scientists that they were, decided after a few experiments that this anointing was against logic since it had never succeeded, and continued to keep their ears open for tales of tiny children whose mothers thought they might have a future on the halls. ¶ Dwarfs do, in fact, generally provide entertainment of a fairly high standard. This is the reason why kings and emperors always liked to have a few around, not only as jesters but as advisers. Dwarfs who combined wit with wisdom were not too hard to find. Like the court jesters whom they superseded – there was a dwarf at the court of Louis XIV of France at a date long after court jesters had been abandoned – dwarfs were permitted unlimited freedom of speech. Accordingly, one of the kings of Denmark made one of his dwarfs prime minister in order to get at truths about the political situation which other men were afraid to utter. ¶ Even after Louis XIV, dwarfs were popular at the papal court in Rome. Cardinal Vitelli stage-managed a banquet there at which the attendants at table were thirty-four dwarfs. Peter the Great of Russia had a passion for dwarfs, and in 1710 gave a great celebration in honour of the marriage of the favourite, Valakoff, with the dwarf of the Princess Prescovy Theodorovna. Subsequently such marriages were forbidden in Russia because of the difficult and dangerous labour which might follow during childbirth. But elsewhere in Victoria's time marriages between dwarfs were neither forbidden nor unknown, nor were marriages between dwarfs and people of normal stature. The child of the marriage between a female dwarf and a physically normal man was born, if not without difficulty, without deformity, and was of normal size, though the face was an extraordinary exaggeration of the mother's, which itself was an exaggeration of a child's head. ¶ The most prolific dwarfs on record were Robert Skinner, height 25 inches, and his wife Judith Skinner, height 26 inches, who between them had fourteen children, all well-formed, healthy, and of normal stature. ¶ The Victorians, having noted that many dwarfs were persons of extraordinary intelligence, pursued the subject, occasionally demonstrating theories that modern scientists cannot sustain. At the Natural History Society of Bonn in 1868 a post-mortem examination was con-

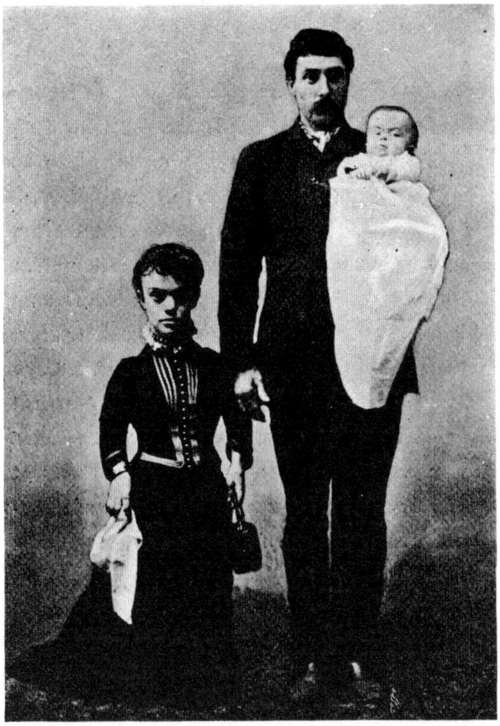

A female dwarf with her husband and child.

ducted on a dwarf who had lived to the age of sixty-one and had been remarkable for his sagacity. Scalpel in hand, Dr Schaufhausen demonstrated that the weight of the dwarf's brain was one-nineteenth of the weight of the body, whereas in a normal subject the proportion would be between one-thirtieth and one-forty-fourth. The weight of the brain he was toying with was 1183.33 grammes, or about 2.6 lb. out of a body weight of 45 lb. But even heavier, compared with the body, might have been the brain of a hydrocephalic idiot with similar stature. ¶ In the nineteenth century there was insufficient statistical evidence to pontificate on the hereditary tendency to produce dwarfism. Cases were noted where a woman was delivered of four dwarfs (but at a time when medical documentation was unreliable). The famous Welsh dwarf Hopkin Hopkins, who died of old age at seventeen weighing only 12 lb., had a sister five years younger who was as small as he was and was also showing signs of senility, but they had four normal brothers and sisters. Virey documented adequately an eight-year-old German dwarf who was only 18 inches tall, the length of a normal new-born infant; and, although the parents of this child were of normal size, they did have another child who was also a dwarf. ¶ There are two instances of great age in dwarfs. In the year of Victoria's accession there died in Durham a Polish gentleman of diminutive stature who had been born ninety-eight years previously, in 1739. He was Joseph Borwilaski, who was famous all over Europe. He became quite a scholar, speaking French and German adequately as well as English. In 1761, at the age of twenty-two, when he was only 28 inches tall, he married a woman of ordinary stature and she bore him two children who were also normal. He was exhibited in many countries but finally settled down in the north of England. Another English dwarf, Mary Jones of Shropshire, who was 32 inches tall but much deformed, died at the age of a hundred. ¶ Richeborg, a dwarf only 23 inches in height, died in Paris in 1858 aged ninety. In childhood he had been a servant of the House of Orleans and had become their pensioner. During the French Revolution he passed in and out of Paris disguised as an infant in a nurse's arms, carrying in his head memorized dispatches which were too dangerous to be set down on paper. ¶ Charles Stratton, whose career as General Tom Thumb has already been noted, was above normal weight when he was born, but he stopped growing when he was about five months old, with a length of 21 inches, and his career as a diminutive started soon afterwards. In spite of the claim that he had kissed a million women in England, his features were said to be anything but inviting. But he had most engaging manners and a truly generous nature. When Barnum, the circus proprietor who had set him on the road to fame, fell upon bad times and Tom Thumb heard about it, it was the General who financed Barnum out of his own savings from his career in show business in order to set Barnum up for another go. Tom's marriage with Lavinia Warren, one of the dwarf sisters Barnum had brought back from England to America, produced one child, Minnie, but she died of cerebral congestion some months after birth. ¶ On Tom Thumb's retire-

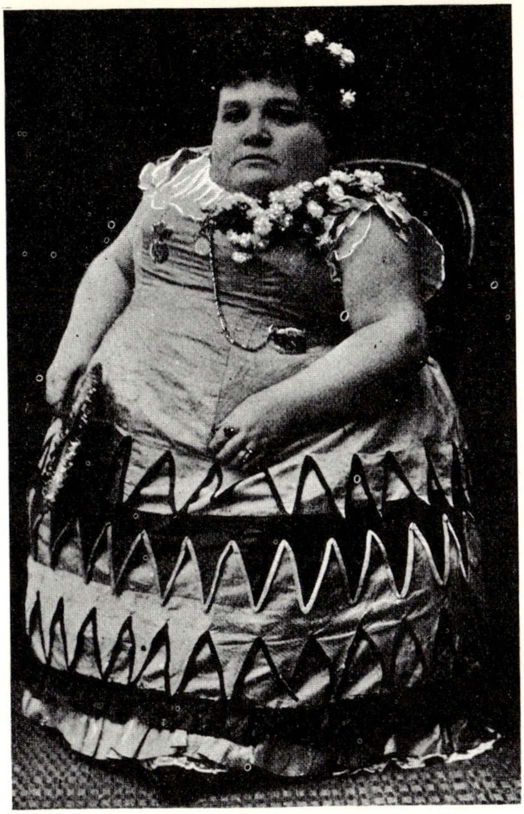

Carrie Akers, 34 inches tall and over 22 stone in weight.

ment, another dwarf called himself General. He was born with the name of Morris, and at a height of 35 inches he married a wife who was even smaller, and toured England with her under the title of 'General and Mrs Small'. Mrs General Small presented the master with twins in 1895, being brought to bed at Blaenavon, North Wales. The youngsters were healthy and of normal stature. ¶ Certainly among the lightest of authenticated Victorian dwarfs was Hattie Moritz, a pretty and delicate young lady who at the age of twenty weighed 36 lb. and was only 22 inches tall. Nearly nine times as heavy was Carrie Akers, who though only 34 inches tall weighed 309 lb., just over 22 stone. She was a victim of the 'Fat Boy' type of hormone deficiency producing gross obesity and presenting itself before the natural growth of youth was completed. ¶ In the days before it could be medically controlled, precocious development in boys and girls of normal

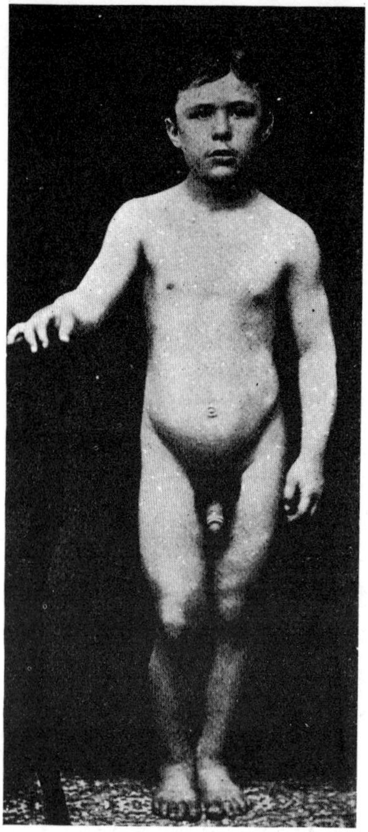

Precocious development in a boy of five years and three months.

stature could on occasion come on with such rapidity that this blatant abnormality caused the onlooker unfamiliar with the case to be unsure whether he was observing an under-developed man or an over-developed boy. This was particularly so when the subject had developed the sexual organs at what could be a truly alarming rate of growth for his or her age. The child of five years and three months with the outstanding apparatus illustrated had, as well as a full growth of pubic hair, a moustache growing on his upper lip which his father was constrained to keep shaving in order not to attract attention to the boy when he was clothed. The lad was just 4 feet tall when the photograph was taken. ¶ Precocious development entailed such a hasty growth that at a very early period in life the subject reached the dimensions of an adult. Often this change was accompanied by the embarrassing side-effects of adolescence without even the partial control which adolescents gradually acquire. But instances were known to the Victorians – who were keenly interested in this subject, since a particular Victorian vice was the deflowering of very young girls, and there was a depraved technical interest in the implications of the onset of puberty and the legal age of consent – where the anomaly of precocious puberty had a definite term of development. After acquiring adult growth at an early age, there was in some subjects an apparent cessation of the development, and the subsequent adult life showed no distinguishing characters. ¶ 'Man-boys', those remarkable male children characterized by early puberty and extraordinary development in infancy, were known in medical manuals and in the literature of curiosa from earliest times. According to Pliny, Euthimedes in Salamis had a son who grew to the equivalent of 4 feet 6 inches in three years; but he was said to have a dull mind, no wit to speak of, besides a dull demeanour and a heavy gait. But his voice had broken by the time he died at three years of age suffering from general debility. The sprightly Craterus, however, brother of King Antigonus, was an infant, a young man, a mature man, an old man, and married and fathered children – all in the space of seven years. *The Philosophical Transactions of the Royal Society of London* mention a boy born at Willingham, near Cambridge, in 1741 who had the external marks of puberty at the age of twelve months, and when he died aged five had the appearance of an old man. He was called *prodigium Willinghamense,* but he was certainly not the only male observed to have a penile erection immediately after birth, since this phenomenon is recorded in many of the older journals. ¶ Very precise measurements were made of young Philip Howarth, who was born at Quebec Mews, Portman Square, London, on 21 February 1806, and within a year had lost his babyish roundness of form and feature, had become pale and awkward and long in his limbs like a growing boy, and was in addition extremely ugly. His penis and testicles increased ominously in size, his voice broke, and pubic hair appeared. At the age of three he was 3 feet 4½ inches tall and weighed 51¼ lb.

The length of his penis when erect was $4\frac{1}{2}$ inches and the circumference 4 inches. His thigh measured $13\frac{1}{2}$ inches round, his waist 24 inches, and his biceps 7 inches. In spite of his unprepossessing looks, he was reported to be clever, very strong, and muscular. ¶ In a review of this aspect of precocious growth published in 1890, six recent cases were cited of early puberty in boys (surprisingly, there was no report of early puberty in girls, although the visible instances of the early formation of breasts would have been more noticeable, easier to check, and, one would have thought, more common, whatever the scruples about reporting early menstruation). One of the boys recorded died at the age of five showing symptoms of premature senility. At the age of twelve months he had shown signs of enlargement of the sexual organs. Another boy was over 3 feet 6 inches tall at the age of three, weighed 50 lb., and had seminal discharges. In another case the boy's voice broke when he was twelve months old, in addition to the other physical demonstrations. One boy aged six was reported who was 4 feet 2 inches tall and weighed 74 lb. His legs were proportionally short, as in a dwarf, and his genitals were as well developed as those of an adult. He had a short, dark moustache, but no hair on his chin, although his pubic hair was thick, black, and curly. He had a deep male voice, and under excitement he discharged semen four or five times a day. ¶ Although the physical condition of these lads often steadied in adult years, so that they did not continue to develop noticeably fast throughout their lives, but merely completed an abnormally hurried rush into manhood, a minority did die of sheer senility in their first years, sometimes as early as the age of five. Mentally, too, they were in bad shape because of the stress entailed in keeping up with their confused and uncertain role in the world. In the *Medical Press and Circular* of London Dr Campbell reported on a case that he had followed for ten years. The lad in question was then aged fourteen. By the time he was fifteen months old this prodigy had hair in the pubic region and his external genitals were abnormally large. At the age of two they were fully developed. But in the following twelve years their size and condition had not materially changed. From time to time during his early years this boy manifested great sexual excitement. From the age of four he had seminal discharges, but before the age of seven no tests had been done to determine whether the semen contained spermatozoa. At fourteen the lad had the muscular development of a man of twenty-five. But his education was markedly defective because, as one indication of his confusion, he had very frequently failed to attend school. ¶ One isolated instance of the most extraordinarily rapid and apparently time-limited growth in a boy – but principally an example of abnormally speedy development which is usually the physical accompaniment of adolescence – is the report Desbois of Paris made in 1888 of a boy of eleven under his care who grew 6 inches in extra height within fifteen days. ¶ Rare and tragic cases were those of congenital asymmetry and hemihypertrophy where one half of the body of a child grows at an abnormal rate while the other continues at a natural progression. The distressing case illustrated was reported by Adams in the *Archives of Pediatrics* of December 1894. The boy was ten at the time the photographs were taken. There was nothing noteworthy in the family history, and he had suffered from none of the diseases of childhood.

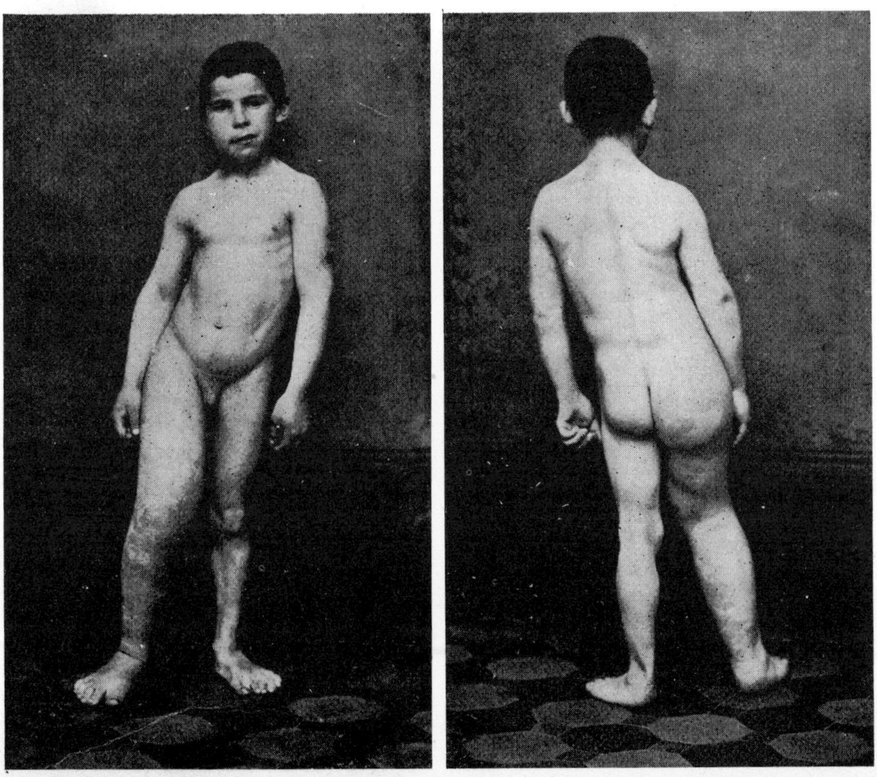

A case of hemihypertrophy.

Some little deformity was noticeable at birth, but not to such a degree as at a later period. The increased growth affected the entire right half of the body, including the face, but was most noticeable in the leg, thigh, and buttock. Numerous telangiectatic spots (surface areas showing a web-like appearance, caused by a number of tortuous dilated capillary blood vessels) were scattered irregularly over the body, but most thickly on the right side, especially on the outer surface of the leg. As would be expected, among other physical anomalies the condition produced a decided limp in the youngster. ¶ In the *Quarterly Medical Journal* of April 1895 Milne reported a case of hemihypertrophy in a girl of twelve months. The only deviation from uniform excess of size on the right side was shown in the forefinger and thumb, which were of the same size as on the other hand. The left side showed no overgrowth of any of its members except a little enlargement of the second toe. At about this time Milne also reported to the Sheffield Medico-Chirurgical Society an instance of unilateral hypertrophy (one-sided excessive growth) in a girl of nineteen months, but he suspected that in addition to an over-development of growth on the right side there was a complicating deficiency of growth on the left. There were six teeth on the right side and one on the left. ¶ Obesity in humans can be general or only partial, as when it occurs on the belly and breasts of both men and women without materially affecting other parts. General obesity in infancy was sometimes known in Victorian medical

LEFT
A thirteen month-old who weighed over 5 stone.

RIGHT
'Baby Chambers'.

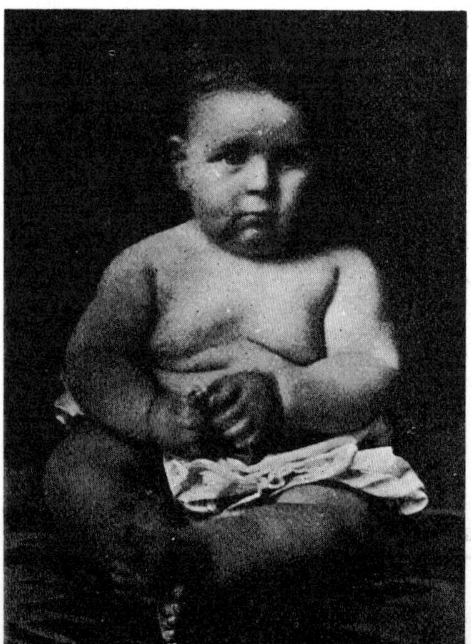

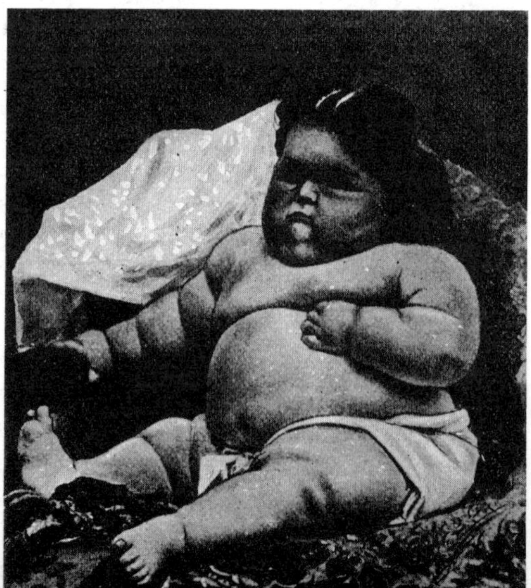

circles as 'congenital corpulency'. Often it was not recognized by mothers in its early stages. The photograph of the thirteen-month-old child might have been innocently entered for a bouncing baby competition. Yet the child weighed 75 lb. (5 stone 5 lb.), which is an unexpected weight to take when lifting a child just over a year old. On the other hand, there could be little doubt in a parent's mind about the marked obesity of another well-known nineteenth-century exhibit of infantile obesity, who was known as 'Baby Chambers'. ¶ Grisolles of Leipzig mentioned a child who was so fat at the age of twelve months that there was constant danger of suffocation. (Miss Conley, a member of an American travelling circus, who weighed 479 lb., or 34 stone 3 lb., was smothered in bed by rolling over on her face; she was unable to turn on her back without help.) The child's story had a happier ending, for she lost all her obesity from the age of two and a half, and in later life was remarkable for her slender figure. The suffering girl in boots weighed 201 lb. when she was nine years old. MacNaughton of New York described Susanna Tripp, who at six years of age weighed 203 lb. and though only 3 feet

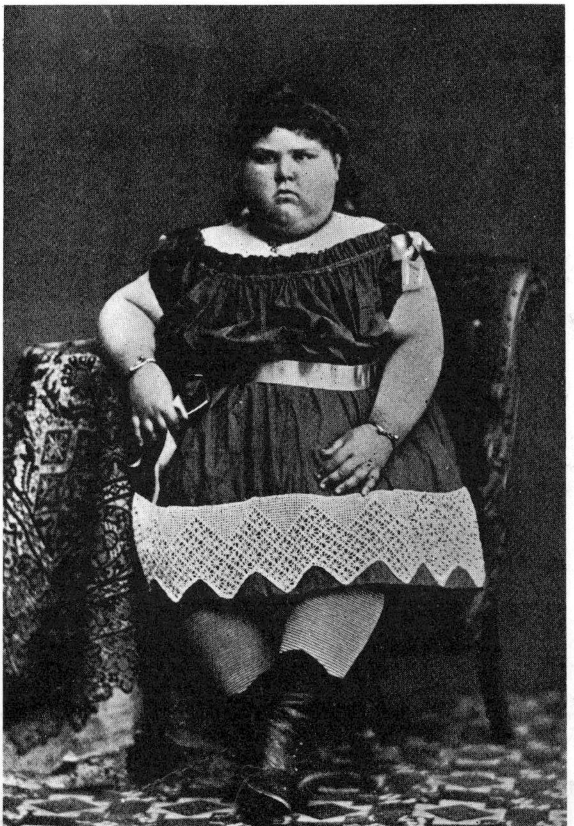

Age nine,
weight 201 pounds.

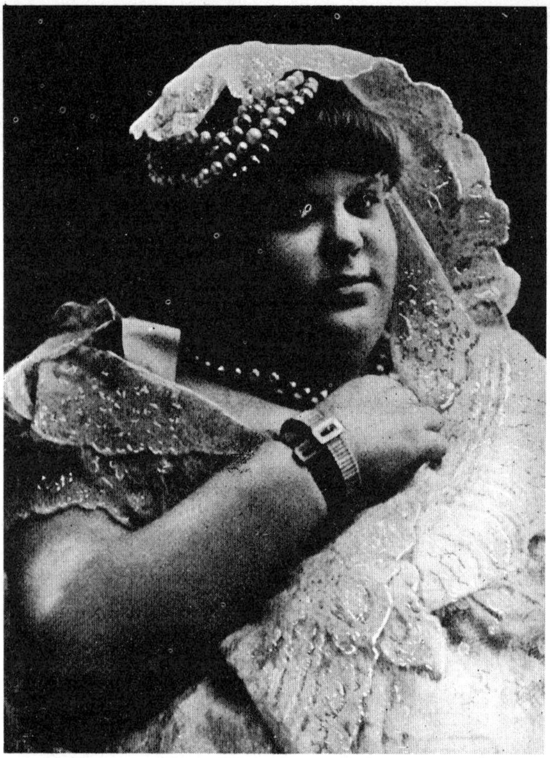

Millie Josephine of Chicago aged 13, weight 422 pounds.

6 inches tall was bigger round the waist, measuring 4 feet 2 inches. Her younger sister Deborah weighed 119 lb. Neither of the two had weighed over 7 lb. at birth, and they both began to grow alarmingly at the fourth month. Millie Josephine, of Chicago, reputed to have been aged thirteen when the photograph was taken, who was exhibited in connection with her appearance in a travelling fair, was 5 feet 6 inches tall and weighed 422 lb. (30 stone 2 lb.). ¶ Victorians noted that it was chiefly in Great Britain and in Holland that the most remarkable instances of obesity were recorded, and the most colossal weights were attained very consistently in Holland. There were, however, some localities where extreme corpulency was considered an adornment of the female sex and was consequently striven for energetically. In 1881 Wartegg reported to Vienna from Tunis that this held for the Jewesses of Tunis, who from the age of ten years were systematically confined in narrow, dark rooms, where they were

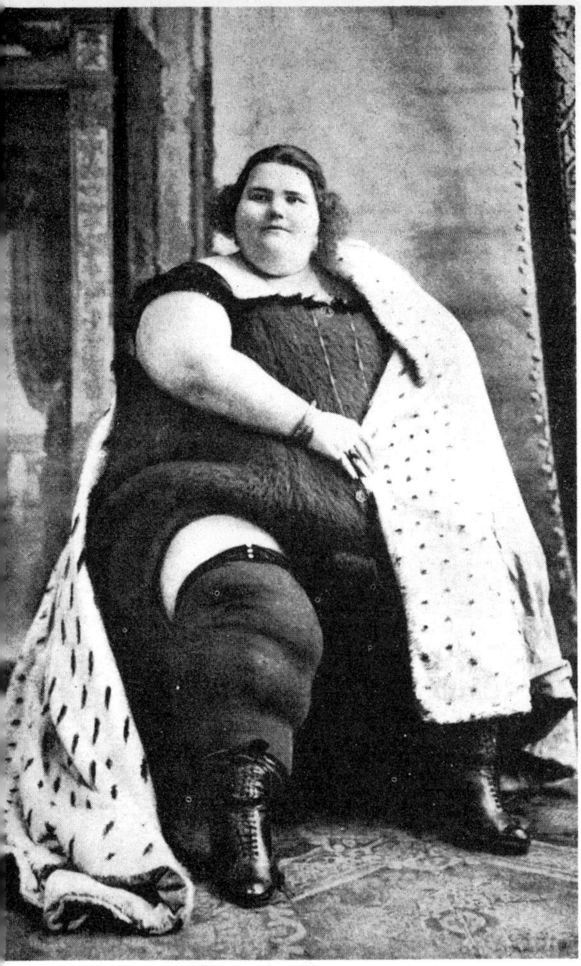

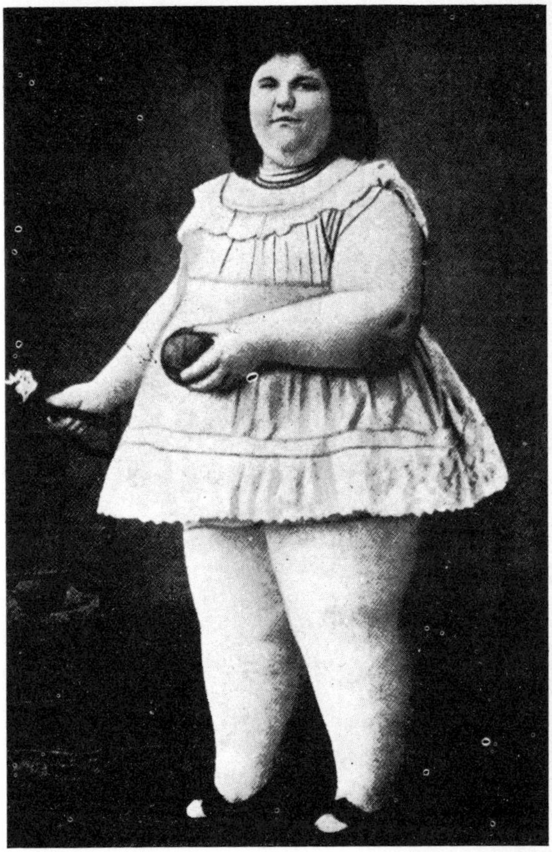

fed on 'farinaceous foods and the flesh of young puppies' until they became almost shapeless masses of fat. At that time the whole of Morocco was weight-watching in the opposite direction to today's trend, and Ebstein reported that the Moorish women reached their desired grossness with astonishing speed by concentrating on a diet of dates and cous-cous. ¶ Fat individuals, especially fat ladies, somewhat naturally graduated into show business in those gawping times. Jenny Letto at least had a grace of symmetry, but as a record-holder she was easily beaten by Teresina, 'Queen Colossus', who weighed 583 lb. (41 stone 9 lb.). When female obesity could be combined with a well-developed beard, naturally the admission price was higher and the financial reward of the exhibitor greater: fat profits that no egalitarian sought very hard to eliminate. ¶ Besides those unfortunate

LEFT

Jenny Letto.

RIGHT

Teresina who weighed 583 pounds.

victims of obesity who were smothered in their sleep, fat people have always been in danger from their propensity to slide into a waking stupor, or half-sleep, while they are sitting up; and to sleep in this position carries an additional risk of suffocation through the relaxing of muscles and the bearing down of weight. There are instances recorded of primitive doctors on constant duty to stick needles in the backs of fat people in order to prevent this fall into sleep while sitting, with its recurring danger of suffocation. But the most famous fat man in England, Daniel Lambert (who was born in Leicester on 13 March 1770), was a remarkably agile person. At about the age of nineteen he realized that he was developing an uncontrollable weight, and he therefore set himself to develop extraordinary strength. By much practice he could easily lift a weight of 500 lb., and he could kick 7 feet high whilst standing on one leg. Eventually he weighed 739 lb. (52 stone 11 lb.), and he was over 9 feet in girth. He had many visitors, one of whom was the dwarf Borwilaski, who was mentioned earlier. Lambert asked the dwarf how much cloth he needed for a suit and was told about three-quarters of a yard, to which he replied that Borwilaski could take home a sleeve from one of his suits, since that would be more than sufficient. ¶ In the *Dictionnaire des sciences médicales* Dupuytren gives the history of Marie-Françoise Clay, the most notorious fat lady of her time. Having achieved the record of being the stoutest woman then known by the age of twenty-five, she married and subsequently had six children. She followed her husband on foot from town to town, in their trade of old-clothes dealers. At the age of forty she was 5 feet 1 inch tall, and one inch larger round the waist. Her head was small and her neck was entirely obliterated. Her breasts were over a yard in circumference, and hung as low as her navel. Her arms hung high, being separated from her body by the fat in her armpits. Her belly was enormous and was augmented by her six pregnancies. Her thighs and haunches were said to be formidable. In her forties she developed an organic heart disease of which, after an interval, she died. There was another woman in Paris who, weighing 486 lb. at the age of twenty-four, could not mount into any cab or omnibus in the city. She was forced to walk, which she found difficult, not so much because of the weight on her feet as because she found it almost impossible to keep her balance as she moved one leg. William Campbell, the landlord of the Duke of Wellington inn in Newcastle-on-Tyne, weighed 728 lb. (52 stone), which he carried better than some because of his height of 6 feet 4 inches. He measured 96 inches round the shoulders, 85 inches round the waist, and 35 inches round the calf. The demolition of his bedroom at his death, when the body had to be lowered three floors by block and tackle, has already been mentioned. The coffin at the funeral weighed fifteen hundred pounds. ¶ There was a famous wine-shop keeper on the quais of Paris who had to use three large chairs when sitting down behind her specially constructed bar. In Switzerland there was a 40-stone man who each day ate five times as much as a normal person. When travelling, he found the greatest difficulty in getting into a railway carriage and usually contented himself by taking possession of the luggage compartment. ¶ The Victorians recognized a condition, which Dercum of Philadelphia called adiposis dolorosa, in which there was excessive obesity but extraordinary additional mental symptoms, a recurrent headache, and a generally painful condition different from the discomfort of massive corpulence. His photographs naturally show the physical presentation of obesity rather than the mental symptoms. Dercum considered it a connective-tissue dystrophy (defective structure, due to shortage of essential factors, of the supporting or packing material of the flesh – a fibrous gel in mucous and other fluids with scattered cells, blood vessels, and nerve fibres). The first case illustrated was an Irish widow who died in her early fifties both alcoholic and syphilitic. Some four years previously her arms had begun to enlarge and this subsequently affected her shoulders. The obesity went on to demonstrate itself in her back and the sides of her chest. The parts affected were elastic, without pitting. In some places the fat was bunched into lobes, in others it appeared as though filled with bundles of worms. The skin was not thickened and the muscles were not involved. In the right

'Adiposis dolorosa':
the Irish widow.

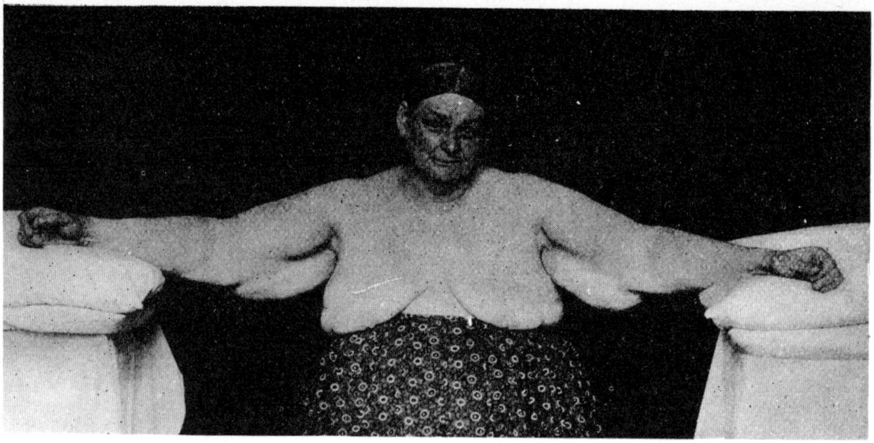

arm there was unendurable pain to the touch, and this condition occurred to a lesser degree in the left arm. In the second case illustrated, a married Englishwoman of sixty-three, the enlarged tissue was said to be very unevenly distributed, though this is not apparent from the photograph, and the occurrence of pain was similar to the previous case. On this woman's death she weighed 300 lb., and the fat over the abdomen was 3 inches thick. In another case the fat below the navel was 7 inches thick, and there was excessive prominence of the mons veneris. ¶ Naturally there were a number of afflictions known which, though counterfeiting general obesity, were due to a more specific cause: elephantiasis; what was then called dropsy – oedema, the collection of an abnormal amount of fluid in the tissues, collected in sites such as the ankles or pulling down soft flesh such as the abdomen; myxoedema, a condition due to under-activity of the thyroid which leads not only to swelling of the limbs and face but also to mental retardation. On the other hand, some aspects of super-obesity can counterfeit more remote serious conditions like the presentation of ovarian cyst. Afflictions of this nature plunge so deeply into the pathetic as well as the grotesque that even the Victorians could not find circus room for them. Yet poverty occasionally forced the sufferers to coax a sore-needed penny for their display. ¶ No such reservations seem to have sabotaged the display of 'human skeletons', of whom J. W. Coffey was the

Victorian prince. Coffey was notorious among all his friends in show business for his hearty appetite and his bouncing good health. This was not the case with another nineteenth-century 'living skeleton', Claude Seurat – no relation of the painter Georges-Pierre and only accidentally, if at all, an inspirer of *pointillisme*. Seurat's daily intake of victuals was of the order of one penny roll and a few sips of wine. His skeleton was plainly visible, with the skin stretched tightly over it. The distance from the chest to the spine was only 3 inches *measured from the outside*. The pulsations of his heart were plainly visible. The circumference of his biceps was only 4 inches. He enjoyed what he took to be good health, and slept well, provided the bed was not too hard. His voice was extremely weak and shrill. ¶ Calvin Edson, another 'living skeleton', had become so in very strange circumstances. As a man of twenty-five he was serving as an American soldier against the British in the War of 1812. After the battle of Plattsburg in 1813 he lay down in the cold in complete exhaustion and became benumbed. He instantly began to lose weight, but did not greatly diminish in strength. Five years later his weight had gone down to 60 lb. from the original 125 lb., but he was in perfect health and could chop a cord of wood without fatigue. He was the father of four children. ¶ In some cases the 'human skeleton' was a living demonstration of extreme muscular atrophy. The successful showground exhibit Rosa Lee Plemons,

[redacted]

It was absolutely unrealistic to display as an extreme of the grotesque the patient pictured with the extraordinary atrophic condition of all the tissues of the body which ought, in a normal human, to have developed through childhood and adolescence. Persons of this type were always sickly and presented all the symptoms of progressive muscular atrophy. They cannot therefore be classed with the true examples of more 'natural' thinness, in which the health is only slightly affected, and in many cases not at all. It is remarkable that the man shown here suffered from non-development of every muscle associated with human growth, so that his head is completely out of proportion to his adult body, in much the same degree as the head of a dwarf. Yet the face is lined and aged, and growth has occurred in it even to the moustache.

CHAPTER FIVE

HUMAN SMELLS, ADDICTIONS, EXTRAORDINARY FEATS

EACH INDIVIDUAL as long as he lives is wrapped around with an odour peculiarly his own, due to exhaled breath, excretions, and above all to unperceived perspiration: this is what the Victorians were taught, and their painstaking researchers compiled libraries of evidence to confirm this and many other human individualities. They believed that the ability to recognize the odour of a separate individual was by no means unknown in civilized society, although they conceded that it was more highly developed in savage tribes. Fournier quoted the instance of a young man with the selectivity of a dog, who in wartime could smell enemy scouts by their scent, and in peacetime used his nose alone to smell out his wife from any other person – no mean feat when performed at the ball before Waterloo. Fournier went on to particularize a French woman living in Naples who had an extreme super-sensitiveness of smell. 'The slightest odor was to her intolerable; sometimes she could not tolerate the presence of certain individuals. She could tell in a numerous circle which women were menstruating. This woman could not sleep in a bed which any one else had made, and for this reason discharged her maid, preparing her own toilet and her sleeping apartments.' De Gassicourt witnessed this particular subject, but in consultation with several of the physicians of Paris could do no more than attribute her excessive sensitiveness to the climate. ¶ Famous in Victorian smoking-rooms was the anecdote about the Hungarian monk mentioned in the *Journal des Savants* who believed that he was able to decide the chastity of females by the sense of smell alone. But the fame which this monk acquired lay more in the versatile uses to which he was said to have put his gift in the corollaries to the original story which were invented with the greatest fluency. ¶ The smell of certain individuals was believed to be stronger than others, and there are many historical references to confirm it. Plutarch wrote in his history that Alexander the Great exhaled an odour similar to that of violets, and his undergarments also smelled profusely of this natural perfume. The smell of sulphur, in modern days more familiar as the basis of the stink bomb, was said to emanate from some people, and, according to Martial, the lady Thais was an example of this class of people, whose odour was insupportable. Schmidt, a medical writer, completed an account of a journeyman saddler of a rather robust constitution whose hands exhaled a smell of sulphur so powerful and penetrating that he rapidly emptied any room in which he happened to be. Dr Rayer was once consulted by a valet de chambre who could never keep a place because of the odour he left behind him in the rooms in which he worked. ¶ Hammond said in the *London Medical Record* that when the blessed Venturni of Bergamons officiated at the altar people struggled to come near him in order to enjoy the odour he exhaled. He added that according to a popular belief St Francis de Paul, after he had subjected himself to frequent disciplinary inflictions including a fast of forty days, exhaled a most perceptible and delicious odour. Hammond attributed the peculiar odours of the saints of earlier days to neglect of washing and, in a measure, to affections of the nervous system. These odours were, of course, augmented, or in some cases cancelled or substituted, by aromatics and incense and other perfumes and deodorants artificially applied. ¶ Brieude classified human smell – that is, the odour emanated rather than the sharpness of the nose – by sex, age, climate, habits, ailments, passions, emotions, and occupations, which all modified the humours exhaled and resulted in necessarily differing odours. According to Brieude, breast-fed infants had a peculiar sourish smell, caused by the butyric acid of the mother's milk, while bottle-fed children smelt like strong butter. After weaning, the odours of babies were deemed to become less decided. Boys reaching puberty were said to exhibit 'peculiar odors which are similar to those of animals when in heat. These odors are leading symptoms of what Borden calls "seminal fever" and are more strongly marked in those of a voluptuous nature. They are said to be caused by the absorption of spermatic fluid into the circulation and its subsequent elimination by the skin. This peculiar circumstance, however, is not seen in girls, in whom menstruation is sometimes to be distinguished by an odor similar to that of leather. Old age produces an odor similar to that of dry leaves, and there have been persons who declared that they could tell approximately the age of individuals by the sense of smell.' ¶ Victorian lore then went on into regions which in later times would have qualified it for castigation on ethnically discriminating grounds: 'Certain tribes and races of people have characteristic odors. Negroes have a rank ammoniacal odor, unmitigated by cleanliness; according to Pruner-Bey it is due to a volatile oil set free by the sebaceous follicles. The Esquimaux and Greenlanders have the odors of their greasy and oily foods, and it is said that the Cossacks, who live much with their horses, and who are principally vegetarians, will leave the atmosphere charged with odors several hours after their passage in numbers through a neighborhood. The lower race of Chinamen are distinguished by a peculiar musty odor which may be noticed in the laundry shops [of English ports and American cities]. Some people, such as the low grade of Indians, have odors, not distinctive, and solely due to the filth of their persons. Food and drink . . . markedly influence the odor of an individual'. ¶ Intercourse could not go unperceived by a Victorian with a keen sense of smell and the correct handbook. Preissmann stated in 1877 that for six hours' after coitus there was a peculiar odour noticeable in the breath, owing to a particular secretion of the buccal glands (in the mouth). This odour was most perceptible in men of about thirty-five, and could be discerned at a distance of from four to six feet. Preissmann added that this fact would be of great medico-legal value in the early arrest of those charged with rape. This anticipation of the breathalyser was complicated by the current belief that immediately after coitus the breath smelt of chloroform, and an authoritative statement appeared in the *Medical Press and Circular* of London in 1863 to the effect that after coitus even naturally foul breath becomes sweet. In those male-chauvinist days no medical attention at all was paid to the breath of women after coitus, but the only practical result can have been that women were thereby put at a great advantage. For even if the seducer could be tracked down and breathalysed, the seductress never could. Joseph might, with a fair policeman and no bribery, get off free or escape with a caution; but Potiphar's wife would never even be charged. ¶ The emotions, according to nineteenth-century scientific belief, had a decided effect on the odour of an individual. Gambrini, quoted by Monin, who wrote a whole treatise entitled *Sur les Odeurs du Corps Humain* in 1885, mentioned a young man, 'unfortunate in love and violently jealous', whose whole body exhaled a sickening, pernicious, and foetid odour. Orteschi met a young lady who exhaled the strong odour of vanilla from the commissures of her fingers (that is, the basins of the spaces between her fingers: 'finger-pits' on the analogy of armpits). ¶ Rayer, who had previously had the odorous manservant to deal with, wrote of a woman under his care at the Hôpital de la Charité who was affected with chronic peritonitis and who for some time before her death exhaled a very decided odour of musk. The smell had been noticed over several days, but was thought to be due to a bag of musk which might have been put purposely into the bed to overpower bad smells.

The woman, however, gave full assurance that she had no kind of perfume about her and that her clothes had been frequently changed. The odour of musk in this case was very perceptible on the arms and other portions of the body, but did not become more powerful by friction. After continuing for about eight days it grew fainter and nearly vanished before the patient's death. Speranza noted a similar case in the *Archives générales de médicine.* ¶ Paré, who was somewhat too credulous to be accepted as a scientific expert, stated that persons with red hair and freckled complexions had a noxious exhalation, that the odour of prussic acid came from dark individuals, and that blonds exhaled a secretion resembling musk. Fat persons, he said, frequently had an oily smell. ¶ Disorders of the nervous system were believed to be associated with peculiar odours. Fèvre said that the smell of lunatics' sweat resembled that of yellow deer or mice, and another alienist, Knight, declared that the absence of this symptom would enable him to tell whether insanity was feigned or not – a facility which surely could have affected few people other than Hamlet. Burrows further bolstered this theory by declaring that in the absence of further evidence he would not hesitate to pronounce a person insane so long as he could smell the odours he already associated with insanity: mice and yellow deer. Sir William Gull and other venereologists declared that they could detect syphilis by smell. Hammond referred to three cases under his notice in which specific odours were the results of affections of the nervous system. One of these cases was a young woman of hysterical tendencies who was perpetually exhaling the odour of violets, and this smell pervaded her apartments. Hammond affirmed that the odour was only given off by the left half of her chest, and he could obtain concentrated samples of it by collecting her perspiration from that part on a handkerchief, heating it over a Bunsen burner with four ounces of spirit, and distilling the resultant mixture. ¶ Hammond also spoke of a young lady subject to chorea (in this context, St Vitus' dance) who quite unconsciously exhaled a perspiration flavoured with the scent of pineapple. A hypochondriac gentleman in his care smelt of violets, while a young woman with the migraine, when she was suffering from an intense sick headache, exhaled an odour resembling Limburger cheese. ¶ Barbier met a case of disordered innervation (inconsistency in the obedience to the brain of nervous impulses or muscular contractions) in an infantry captain, the upper part of whose body was subject to such offensive perspiration that despite all treatment he had finally to resign his commission. But an overpowering bad smell is not an uncommon quality and it was met in the most noble families. Henry of Navarre, King Henri IV of France, was a victim of bromidrosis (offensive sweating, particularly from the feet) so that proximity to him was said to be insufferable to his courtiers, and to his many mistresses, who affirmed that his odour was like that of carrion. When his second wife, Marie de' Medici, was preparing for her bridal night, she perfumed her apartments and her person with the essences of the flowers of her own country in order that she might be spared something of the disgusting odour of her spouse, and be reminded a little of home. ¶ To carry the smell of a corpse may be a dangerous property. In lethargy and catalepsy (periods of trance or deep sleep when the limbs will not move from any position in which an observer places them) the perspiration was believed to have very often a cadaverous odour and this led to a number of mistaken diagnoses of death. Schaper and de Meara spoke of some persons retaining the smell of corpses all their life. Doctors maintained that the breath of any of their colleagues who had recently performed a prolonged post-mortem examination smelt for some hours of the odour of the body. ¶ Diseases were said to have their different odours, often, of course, uniting in the so-called 'hospital smell' which was a combination of the exhalations of the individual's skin and the general master-odour of excreta and its masking disinfectants which were the reserve of the hospital. Gout and cholera were supposed to have their own odours. The old scourge typhus diffused an aroma of honey. In diabetes there was the marked odour of apples. The sweat in dysentery bore unmistakably the odour of the body's refuse. The hair too had its peculiar odours, differing in individuals. The hair of the Chinese was said to have an odour of musk which could not be washed away by the strongest of chemicals. The distinctive smell of a woman was thought to be often due to the odour of great masses of hair, in those days when hair could come in luxuriant masses. It was said that wig-makers could tell by the smell whether hair had been cut from a living head or whether it had come from combings, since hair lost its smell when it fell out. In the paroxysms of hystero-epilepsy the hair was said to have a specific odour of urine. Tapeworm infection gave the scalp an odour resembling that of cat's urine. ¶ The Victorians were aware of the sexual fetishism displayed in a perverted taste for the odours of handkerchiefs, shoes, underclothing, and other articles of dress worn by the opposite sex. Harking back to the days of chivalry, Binet maintained that the favours given by fair ladies to medieval knights going into battle or tournament were not only tokens of remembrance and appreciation, but sexual excitants as well. In his work *Osphrésiologie* Cloquet drew attention to the sexual pleasure aroused by the odours of flowers, and told how the duc de Richelieu 'excited his sexual functions' by living in an atmosphere pervaded by these perfumes. In the Orient the nineteenth-century harems were heavily perfumed with extracts and flowers, in accordance with the strong belief in the aphrodisiac effect of these odours and essences. ¶ In his *Psychopathia Sexualis* Krafft-Ebing, who lived for less than the length of Victoria's reign, quoted several interesting cases in which, he wrote, 'the connection between the olfactory and the sensual functions is strikingly verified. The case of Henry III [of France] shows that contact with a person's perspiration may be the exciting cause of passionate love. At the betrothal feast of the King of Navarre and Margaret of Valois he accidentally dried his face with a garment of Maria of Cleves which was moist with her perspiration. Although she was the bride of the Prince of Condé, Henry immediately conceived such a passion for her that he could not resist it, and, as history shows, made her very unhappy. An analogous instance is related of Henry IV, whose passion for the beautiful Gabrielle is said to have originated at the instant when, at a ball, he wiped his brow with her handkerchief.' (Since the Henry IV mentioned here is the Henri IV already noted above with the remarkably overpowering sweaty feet, one suspects that Krafft-Ebing did not know about this king's basic problem.) ¶ Krafft-Ebing continued in *Psychopathia Sexualis:* 'One learns from reading the work of Ploss [*Das Weib*] that attempts to attract a person of the opposite sex by means of the perspiration may be discerned in many forms in popular psychology. In reference to this a custom is remarkable which holds among the natives of the Philippine Islands when they become engaged. When it becomes necessary for the engaged pair to separate they exchange articles of wearing apparel, by means of which each becomes assured of faithfulness. These objects are carefully preserved, covered with kisses, and smelled.' ¶ The love of perfumes manifested by Victorian libertines and prostitutes, as well as 'sensual women of the higher classes', was considered to be very marked and highly significant. Heschl reported a case of a man of forty-five in whom absence of the olfactory sense was associated with imperfect development of the genitals. Garnier collected a number of observations of fetishism in individuals who took sexual satisfaction from the odours of shoes, night-dresses, bonnets, drawers, menstrual napkins, and other objects of the female toilet. He also mentioned 'creatures who have gloated over the odors of the blood and excretions from the bodies of women' and gave the first instances of fetishism among persons who had been arrested in Paris for clipping the long hair from young girls. ¶ Krafft-Ebing stated the obvious facts that animals of both sexes are drawn to each other by the sense of smell, and that almost all animals at the time of rutting emit a very strong odour from their genitals. The dog is thus attracted to the bitch from several miles away. Certain animals such as the musk-ox, civet-cat, and beaver possess glands on their sexual organs that secrete materials having a very strong odour. Musk, a substance possessing the most penetrating odour, was obtained from the preputial follicles (associated with the foreskin of penis or clitoris) of the musk-deer of Tibet, and castor, a substance less penetrating, was obtained from the preputial sacs of the beaver. ¶ The Victorians noted anomalies of human secretions – from abnormally coloured saliva to milk coming from the nipples of men. The coloured saliva was generally traced to some chemical substance that had been trapped by the teeth. Among abnormal modes of exit of urine were mentioned its excretion from the nipples, the eyes, the mouth, the ears, and the navel. There were complicated pathological reasons for most of these occurrences when they were substantiated, which was not always. A case of discharge of urine from the stomach, by vomiting, was typical of a number studied, and in most cases of the anomalous exit of urine a cause was established of congenital malformations or fistulous connections – a fistula being an abnormal connection between two body cavities. ¶ Although older writers had spoken of instances of the abnormal exit of semen, typically through the skin as a sort of perspiration – and this was especially supposed to be the case in satyriasis (excessive sexual desire in the male), in which the semen was believed to be so over-abundant that it escaped by any possible exit – nevertheless Victorian doctors discounted these theories, relying on the fact that they already recognized the smell of semen as a distinct personal odour in certain individuals, and they had no evidence to label these men as putative satyrs. ¶ Coloured sweat had been mentioned by many authorities, the colours exuded ranging from black through various shades of green to violet – and a Nuremberg publication of 1727 even recorded phosphorescent perspiration. Sweat has been said to be sweet after the subject has eaten honey, and in certain circumstances described by Thomas Bartholinus it has tasted like wine. Sir Benjamin Brodie, writing in the *Medico-Chirurgical Transactions* of London in 1845, communicated the history of a young woman on whose face there was a black secretion. When she tried to remove it by washing she was caused great pain. The quantity removed at one time by soap and water was sufficient to make four basins of water as black as if they had had Indian ink poured into them. Brodie thought the condition was analogous to melanosis (a condition in which there are black spots in the tissues). Eventually the secretion on the face and forehead went away, but what followed was the ejection of a similar substance from the bowel, stomach, and kidney, by excretion and vomiting. The secretion was more abundant during the night, and at one time there was an eruption of erysipelas (an acute streptococcal infection of the skin). Eventually the condition was completely cured, but Brodie could give no factual explanation for it. ¶ Once the nineteenth-century doctors began to admit the occurrence of coloured sweat they reported actual findings much more often – frequently in association with chronic sluggish action of the bowels – and produced a whole range of hues: black, brown, yellow, green, and blue. Conradi reported a case of blue perspiration on one half of the scrotum only. This localization was fairly commonly noted with ordinary sweating, especially in cases of hyperidrosis (excessive sweating), where the sweating was variously reported as confined to the right side of the face and scalp, to the whole of the body above the waist but never below, or to a bald spot on a man's head. In the *Medical and Physical Journal* of London (25 February 1885) Myrtle related the case of a man of seventy-seven who began to sweat profusely and continued to do so until he died of exhaustion after three months. Excessive sweating confined to the hands and the feet was deemed, after analysis of many reports from doctors, to be a fairly common occurrence. ¶ The saying that, after an intense effort, one had 'sweated blood' to achieve a particular purpose was well known in Victorian times, and there were instances of its having actually occurred. Because the Bible said that Christ, during his agony in the garden of Gethsemane, had broken out in a bloody sweat – 'His sweat was', according to Luke, 'as it were great drops of blood falling down to the ground' – there were always a few religious zealots who managed to duplicate this process in the extreme of their sympathetic emotion. But instances were recorded in which fear and deep emotions of that nature had caused a sweating of blood. Paullini saw a sailor, terrified during a storm at sea, fall to the deck in a faint at the height of the storm and sweat from his entire body a red perspiration which stained his clothes. He also mentions a bloody sweat following coitus. A number of writers record not only bloody sweat, but also bloody tears, issuing at moments of crisis, particularly when a man was seriously threatened with death or, on a number of occasions, just before his actual execution. ¶ The occurrence of the stigmata, the duplication of the wounds which Christ suffered at the crucifixion, is an area which lay people have regarded with deep reserve, and the Roman Catholic Church itself (for, peculiarly enough, there are no records of the occurrence within any Reformed church) has regarded with more than reserve, with the utmost suspicion of the Devil's Advocate lest the bearer of the stigmata should lay claim to sainthood. The following account, written by Gray from observations made in 1869, is the best-verified Victorian document on the endurance of stigmata, carried, it should be noticed, not only on the trunk and the hands, as was more common, but also on the feet. In other cases of stigmata there has been confusion, and even omission, regarding the site of bleeding from the feet, which can be explained by the fact that, if complete personal, spiritually visual, and ultimately self-hypnotic participation is to be considered, there is much less clarity about the actual position of the wounds, owing to doubts as to whether Christ's feet were crossed or separated on the shaft of the cross. ¶ The study was made of Louise Lateau of Bois d'Haine, a village in Belgium. In 1869 she was twenty-three years old, and her previous life had offered nothing remarkable. Gray wrote:

One Friday Louise Lateau noticed that blood was flowing from one side of her chest, and this recurred every Friday. On each Thursday morning an oval surface about one inch in length on the back of each hand became pink in color and smooth, whilst a similar oval surface on the palm of each hand became of the same hue, and on the upper surface of each foot a pinkish-white square appeared. Examined under a magnifying glass, the epidermis appeared at first without solution [meaning here, interruption] of continuity and delicate. About noon on Thursday a vesicle [blister] formed on the pink surfaces containing clear serum. In the night between Thursday and Friday, usually between midnight and one o'clock, the flow of blood began, the vesicle first rupturing. The amount of blood lost during the so-called stigmata period varied, and some observers estimated it at about one and three-quarter pints. The blood itself was of a reddish color, inclining to violet, about the hue, therefore, of capillary blood, coagulating in the usual way, and the white and red corpuscles being normal in character and relative proportion. The flow ceased on Saturdays. During the flow of blood the patient was in a rapt, ecstatic condition. The facial expression was one of absorption and far-off contemplation, changing often to melancholy, terror, to an attitude of prayer or contrition. The patient herself stated that at the beginning of the ecstasy she imagined herself surrounded by a brilliant light; figures then passed before her, and the successive scenes of the crucifixion were panoramically progressive. She saw Christ in person – His clothing, His wounds, His crown of thorns, His cross – as well as the Apostles, the holy women, and the assembled Jews. During the ecstasy the circulation of the skin and heart was regular, although at times a sudden flush or pallor overspread the face, according with the play of the expression. From midday of Thursdays, when she took a frugal meal, until eight o'clock on Saturday mornings the girl took no nourishment, not even water, because it was said she did not feel the want of it and could not retain anything upon her stomach. During this time the ordinary secretions were suspended.

¶ A completely contrasting instance of the extrusion of blood is the report in the Berlin *Magazin für die gesammte Heilkunde* of a male patient who once or twice a day was attacked with swelling of the scrotum, which at length acquired a deep red colour and a stony hardness, at which time the blood would spring from a hundred points and flow in the finest streams until the scrotum was again empty. ¶ Even more remarkable is the 1835 report in the *Gazette médicale de Paris* of the secretion of maternal milk from the scrotum of a man of twenty-one. The scrotum was tumefied, and to the touch gave the sensation of a human breast, and the parts were pigmented similar to an engorged breast. Analysis showed the secretion to have been true human milk. ¶ The accounts of anomalies in lactation include reports of a wide variety of colour – black, red, green, and yellow. It was accepted that substances previously taken by the mother could affect the quality of the milk – the yellow milk was ascribed to a previous excess of rhubarb. There is one singular case on record, in the Paris *Journal de médicine,* in which a child was poisoned from the milk of its mother after she had been bitten by a snake. ¶ There were also a number of nineteenth-century accounts of metastasis, in which the milk was delivered by ducts other than the breast. Bourdon in the *Journal des Sçavans* mentions milk coming from the thigh, labia, and vulva. Klein in the *London Medical Gazette* speaks of the metastasis of milk to the lochia, the vaginal discharge after childbirth. Gardane in the *Journal de santé* reported metastasis to the lungs, and there was another case on record where this phenomenon caused asphyxia. There is a report of a woman who suffered metastasis of milk to the stomach, and who, with convulsive action of the chest and abdomen, vomited it daily. A peculiar instance of milk in a tumour is that of a Mrs Reed, reported in the *Boston Medical Journal and Record,* who when pregnant with twins developed an abdominal tumour from which 25 lb. of milk were drawn off. ¶ Cases of lactation in the newly-born were well known. In the *Dublin Medical Press* in 1835 Battersby described a male child, three weeks old, whose breasts were full of a fluid which on analysis proved to be human milk. Darby followed this case in the same journal with a record of a child eight days old whose breasts were so engorged that the nurse had to milk it. Variot stated that out of thirty-two children of both sexes, aged from six to nine months, all but six showed the presence of milk in the breasts. ¶ There were also examples of precocious lactation, and lactation in adults without pregnancy. Baudelocque wrote of a girl of eight who suckled her brother with her extraordinarily developed breasts. This child was brought to Paris and milked her breasts in the presence of the Royal Academy. In 1856 Dix, of the Derby Infirmary, reported in the *Medical Times and Gazette* two females whom he had observed with continued lactation although they had never been pregnant. The first was a chaste female of twenty-five, who for two years had abundant and spontaneous discharge of milk. The other was a prostitute of twenty who had never been pregnant but who had for several months an abundant secretion of milk. Zoologists knew that a non-pregnant bitch could secrete milk in abundance. ¶ Lactation in old women was also known. Sir Hans Sloane described a lady of sixty-eight who, though she had not borne a child for twenty years, nursed her grandchildren one after the other. Montegre described a woman in Charente who bore twin sons. Not having enough milk for both, and being too poor to engage a wet-nurse, in desperation she sought the help of a widow named Laverge, sixty-five years old, whose husband had been dead for twenty-nine years. This old woman gave the breast to one of the children, and in a few days an abundant flow of milk was present. For twenty-two months she nursed this boy, who not only thrived but grew into a stronger child than his brother. ¶ Prolonged lactation extending through several pregnancies was also known. In the *New York Journal of Medicine* Green reported a woman of forty-seven, the mother of four children, who after each weaning had so much milk constantly in her breasts that it had to be drawn until the next birth. The classic case was that described by Gomez Pamo in the *Louisville Medical News* (4 August 1883), of a woman in whom lactation seemed indefinitely prolonged. She had married at sixteen, soon became pregnant, and after delivery had continued lactation for over a year without any sign of returning menstruation. She again became pregnant, weaned her first child, and nursed the other without any delay or complication. This occurrence took place fourteen times. She nursed all her first thirteen children up to the time that she found herself pregnant again, and during all pregnancies after the first the flow of milk never entirely ceased. The milk was abundant and of good quality. This report appeared seven years after the birth of her last child, whom she had weaned at the age of two, and not only had menstruation never occurred, but the milk had continued to flow. For the last five years it had not been taken by a child, and on occasion its persistence had been so abundant that it had been necessary to express it from the breasts to relieve painful tension. ¶ With regard to profuse flow of milk at a single childbirth, Remy was quoted in the London *Medical Times and Gazette* as having seen a young woman in Japan from whom $12\frac{1}{2}$ pints of milk were taken every day. This was considered the most extreme case of continued galactorrhea on record. ¶ Gynae-

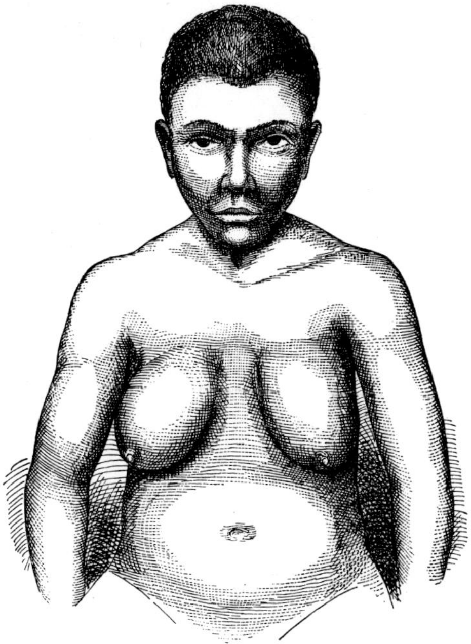

A man with fully-developed breasts.

comastia, the enlargement of a male breast to female proportions, had been spoken of by all medical men since ancient times, but E. Laurent made the most exhaustive study of it, in *Les bisexués, gynécomastes et hermaphrodites*, published in 1894. A sketch from a photograph of one of his subjects is illustrated. The breasts of this man measured 30 centimetres in circumference at the base and hung pendulously like those of a nursing woman. Schuchardt collected 272 cases of gynaecomastia. In a certain number there was feminization in the male characteristics, and Hutchinson reported in the *Archives of Surgery* a number of examples where the external genital organs decreased in proportion to the size of the breast, and the manners became effeminate. Occasionally the presence of only one ultra-developed breast in a man was mentioned. In 1875 Moran communicated to the *Lancet* his examination of a seaman of twenty-one who was admitted to the Royal Naval Hospital at Hong Kong, and whose right breast was as well developed as in a full-grown woman. It had a large brown areola but the nipple was the same size as that of the left breast. The sailor said that he had first noticed the enlargement of the breast when he was sixteen and a half years old, and since that

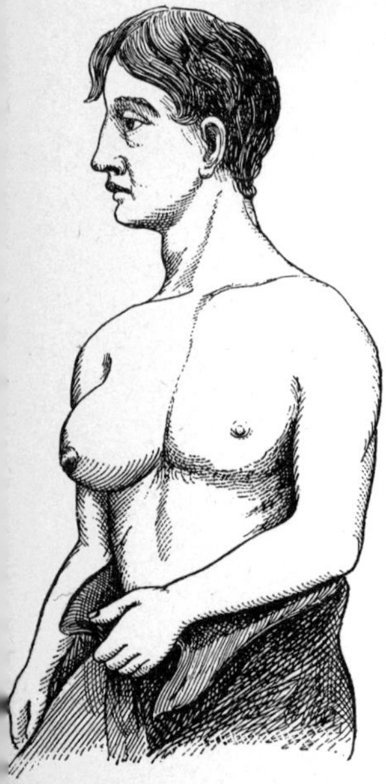

Abnormal development of the right breast in a young man.

time it had steadily grown. No milk was obtainable at any time from the nipple. The external genital organs were well and fully developed. The sailor had no complaint of pain or discomfort from the breast except when he was on duty aloft and had to descend in the usual hurry, when his breast was burnt from contact with the ropes down which he was sliding. ¶ Instances of gynaecomastia were especially interesting when the individuals concerned displayed an ability to suckle babies. A number of cases of this nature were quoted. One concerned another sailor, who after the loss of his wife took his son to his own breast to quieten him, and after three or four days was able to nourish him. According to Mehliss some missionaries in Brazil in the sixteenth century asserted that there was an entire Indian nation there whose women had small and withered breasts and whose children were brought up from birth by suckling the males. Certainly the American Professor Hall exhibited to his class at Baltimore a Negro then aged fifty-five who had suckled all his mistress's family. This man was examined by Dunglison, who reported that the breasts projected 7 inches from the chest, though the external male genital organs were well developed. ¶ There was no grotesque condition that did not interest Victorian medical men. They explored bulimia, the morbid craving for food which in some cases caused the sufferers to consume up to forty pounds of food a day. They researched polydipsia, or abnormal thirst, and recounted the classic stories of people who had to take up to twelve gallons of liquid a day and who, when in dire straits at night, would raise their own chamber-pots to their lips. They amassed the details of perverted appetites, which were often of so sickening a nature that they had even to be barred from elaboration in the smoking-room. They were naturally interested in cannibalism, which in their time was widely practised, though not openly in their own civilization. The explorer H. M. Stanley came back from Africa and declared that there were thirty million inhabitants in the Congo basin alone who relished human flesh above all other meat. ¶ 'The black natives of Australia', Victorians were authoritatively told, 'are all professed cannibals.

Dr. Carl Lumholtz, a Norwegian scientist, spent many months in studying them in the wilds of the interior. He was alone among these savages, who are extremely treacherous. Wearing no clothing whatever, and living in nearly every respect as monkeys do, they know no such thing as gratitude, and have no feeling that can properly be termed human. Only fear of the traveler's weapons prevented them from slaying him, and more than once he had a narrow escape. One of the first of them whom he employed looked more like a brute than a man. "When he talked," says the doctor, "he rubbed his belly with complacency, as if the sight of me made his mouth water." This individual was regarded with much respect by his fellows because of his success in procuring human flesh to eat. These aborigines say that the white man's flesh is salt and occasions nausea. A Chinaman they consider as good for eating as a black man, his food being chiefly vegetable. ¶ 'The most horrible development of cannibalism among the Australian blacks is the eating of defunct relatives. When a person dies there follows an elaborate ceremony, which terminates with lowering of the corpse into the grave. In the grave is a man not related to the deceased, who proceeds to cut off the fat adhering to the muscles of the face, thighs, arms, and stomach, and passes it around to be swallowed by some of the near relatives. All those who have eaten of the cadaver have a black ring of charcoal powder and fat drawn around the mouth. The order in which the mourners partake of their dead relatives is duly prescribed. The mother eats of her children and the children of their mother. A man eats of his sister's husband and of his brother's wife. Mothers' brothers, mothers' sisters, sisters' children, mothers' parents, and daughters' children are also eaten by those to whom the deceased person stands in such relation. But the father does not eat of his children, nor the children of their sire. ¶ 'The New Zealanders, up to very recent times, were probably the most anthropophagous [cannibalistic] race that ever existed. As many as 1000 prisoners have been slaughtered by them at one time after a successful battle, the bodies being baked in ovens underground. If the individual consumed had been a redoubtable enemy they dried his head as a trophy and made flutes of his thigh bones. ¶ 'Among the Monbuttos of Africa human fat is commonly employed for a variety of purposes. The explorer Schweinfurth speaks of writing out in the evenings his memoranda respecting these people by the light of a little oil-lamp contrived by himself, which was supplied with some questionable-looking grease furnished by the natives. The smell of this grease, he says, could not fail to arouse one's worst suspicions against the negroes. According to his account the Monbuttos are the most confirmed cannibals in Africa. Surrounded as they are by a number of peoples who are blacker than themselves, and who, being inferior to them in culture, are held in contempt, they carry on expeditions of war and plunder which result in the acquisition of a booty especially coveted by them – namely, human flesh. The bodies of all foes who fall in battle are distributed on the field among the victors, and are prepared by drying for transportation. The savages drive their prisoners before them, and these are reserved for killing at a later time. During Schweinfurth's residence at the Court of Munza it was generally understood that nearly every day a little child was sacrificed to supply a meal for the ogre potentate. For centuries past the slave trade in the Congo Basin has been conducted largely for the purpose of furnishing human flesh to consumers. Slaves are sold and bought in great numbers for market, and are fattened for slaughter. ¶ 'The Mundurucus of the Upper Amazon, who are exceedingly ferocious, have been accused of cannibalism. It is they who preserve human heads in such a remarkable way. When one of their warriors has killed an enemy he cuts off the head with his bamboo knife, removes the brain, soaks the head in a vegetable oil, takes out bones of the skull, and dries the remaining parts by putting hot pebbles inside of it. At the same time care is taken to preserve all the features and the hair intact. By repeating the process with the hot pebbles many times the head finally becomes shrunken to that of a small doll, though still retaining its human aspect, so that the effect produced is very weird and uncanny. Lastly, the head is decorated with brilliant feathers, and the lips are fastened together by a string, by which the head is suspended from the rafters of the council-house.' ¶ It is remarkable to consider that, less than a century ago, anecdotes of this nature were common gossip in the Travellers' Club. Other explorers came back with tales of the extreme endurance practised in the fire dances of the Navajo Indians. But endurance, to either heat or cold, was a practical subject for research in a milieu of intense exploration without the scientific aids and insulated clothing which are available today. It was as important to know the limits of resistance to cold as to heat. The Victorians had to get used to both, or pay their own people to get used to them. They knew that the Eskimo and other inhabitants of the extreme north could endure for a time a temperature of −60° Fahrenheit, while some of the people inhabiting equatorial regions were apparently healthy at a temperature as high as 130°, and moreover they worked in the sun where the temperature was much higher. In the engine rooms of some steamers plying in tropical waters temperatures as high as 150° were registered, yet the engineers and stokers became used to this heat and worked in it without apparent suffering. The upper classes made experiments in Turkish baths, where it was said that, by progressively exposing themselves to escalating temperatures, people had been able to endure a heat considerably above boiling point, though they had to protect their persons from the furniture, floors, and walls of these rooms. They told each other that the hot air in these baths was intensely dry, so that profuse perspiration was provoked. The Victorians reminded themselves that Sir Joseph Banks, the naturalist and explorer who went round the world with Captain Cook and was also an expert on the colder countries of Newfoundland and Iceland, had gone into training for tropical travel by remaining for some time in a room with a temperature of 211° Fahrenheit, one degree below boiling point. And, they said, his own temperature had never mounted above normal. ¶ Consequently Victorians took more than an academic interest in the so-called 'human salamanders' of the day – the showmen who claimed a particular ability to endure intense heats and survive. Martinez, called 'the French Salamander' though he was born in Havana, had become used to high temperatures through starting life as an apprentice baker. But it took far more exhaustive training and a peak of endurance for him to register his greatest feat. This was to stay inside an oven specially erected in the middle of the Tivoli Gardens in Copenhagen for fourteen minutes when the temperature of the oven was 338°F. His pulse on entering was 70 and on coming out was 130. He often duplicated this feat before enormous assemblies of (paying) spectators, but the temperature of the oven never even approached this furnace at the Tivoli. The rival of Martinez was Chamouni, 'the Russian Salamander', who assumed the title of 'The Incombustible' – but sadly proved that it was an ill-chosen boast. His great feat was to enter an oven with a raw leg of mutton, and not to come out until the meat was well baked. But one day, in the course of this performance, Chamouni did not come out alive. He, too, was roasted. His ashes were conveyed to his native town where a monument was erected over them. ¶ The Victorians were also keenly interested in accounts of savage ceremonies of fire-worship which still existed in their world. An American report ran:

The most remarkable ceremonial of fire worship that survives in this country is practised by the Navajos. They believe in purification by fire, and to this end they literally wash themselves in it. The feats they perform with it far exceed the most wonderful acts of fire-eating and fire-handling accomplished by civilized jugglers. In preparation for the festival a gigantic heap of dry wood is gathered from the desert. At the appointed moment the great pile of inflammable brush is lighted and in a few moments the whole of it is ablaze. Storms of sparks fly 100 feet or more into the air, and ashes fall about like a shower of snow. The ceremony always takes place at night and the effect of it is both weird and impressive. ¶ Just when the fire is raging at its hottest a whistle is heard from the outer darkness and a dozen warriors, lithe and lean, dressed simply in narrow white breech-cloths and moccasins and daubed with white earth so as to look like so many living statues, come bounding through the entrance to the corral that incloses the flaming heap. Yelping like wolves, they move slowly toward the fire, bearing aloft slender wands tipped with balls of eagle-down. Rushing around the fire, always to the left, they begin thrusting their wands toward the fire, trying to burn off the down from the tips. Owing to the intensity of the heat this is difficult to accomplish. One warrior dashes wildly toward the fire and retreats; another lies as close to the ground as a frightened lizard, endeavoring to wriggle himself up to the fire; others seek to catch on their wands the sparks that fly in the air. At last one by one they all succeed in burning the downy balls from the wands. The test of endurance is very severe, the heat of the fire being so great. ¶ The remarkable feats, however, are performed in connection with another dance that follows. This is heralded by a tremendous blowing of horns. The noise grows louder and louder until suddenly ten or more men run into the corral, each of them carrying two thick bundles of shredded cedar bark. Four times they run around the fire waving the bundles, which are then lighted. Now begins a wild race around the fire, the rapid running causing the brands to throw out long streamers of flames over the hands and arms of the dancers. The latter apply the brands to their own nude bodies and to the bodies of their comrades in front. A warrior will seize the flaming mass as if it were a sponge, and, keeping close to the man he is pursuing, will rub his back with it as if bathing him. The sufferer in turn catches up with the man in front of him and bathes him in flame. From time to time the dancers sponge their own backs with the flaming brands. When a brand is so far consumed that it can no longer be held it is dropped and the dancers disappear from the corral. The spectators pick up the flaming bunches thus dropped and bathe their own hands in the fire. ¶ No satisfactory explanation seems obtainable as to the means by which the dancers in this extraordinary performance are able to escape injury. Apparently they do not suffer from any burns. Doubtless some protection is afforded by the earth that is applied to their bodies.

¶ Another favourite topic which had more current interest then than now because of the tales brought back by explorers was that of the so-called 'Wolf Children'. What Victorians wanted to know was: to what extent will a human being resemble a beast when it is deprived of all association with man? ¶ The *Lancet* took this topic up, and made an analysis of six known cases from India where wolves had nurtured small children in their dens. The children were all boys. In one instance the lad was traced from the moment he was carried off by a lurking wolf while his parents were working in the fields, to the time when, having been recovered by his mother six years later, he escaped from her into the jungle. In all these cases certain marked features occurred. In the first, the boy was very inoffensive, except when teased, and then he growled surlily. He would eat anything thrown to him, but preferred meat, which he devoured with canine voracity. He drank a pitcher of buttermilk at one gulp, and could not be induced to wear clothing, even in the coldest weather. He showed the greatest fondness for bones, and gnawed them contentedly, after the manner of his adoptive parents. This child had coarse features, a repulsive countenance, was filthy in his habits, and could not articulate a word. ¶ In another case the child was kidnapped at three and recovered at nine. He muttered, but could not articulate. As in the other case, he could not be enticed to wear clothes. From constantly being on all fours, the front of his knees and his elbows had become hardened. In the third case the father identified a son who had been carried away at the age of six and was found four years afterwards. The intellectual deterioration was not so marked. The boy understood signs, and his hearing was exceedingly acute. When directed by movements of the hands to help the peasants turn out the cattle, he readily understood what was being asked of him. Yet this lad, who must have been of an age when he was talking before he was taken away, could not talk later, nor utter any decidedly articulate sound. ¶ The full reference for this interesting résumé in the *Lancet* is Vol. I of 1888, p. 593. The original paper collecting the cases of wolf-children was said to have been written by Colonel Sleeman, an officer who had served for many years in the Indian forests, and a copy should still be with the British Museum. ¶ A further case of a wolf-child was reported from the Etwah district of India, near the banks of the river Jumna. Again the child was restored to his parents, who found him very difficult to manage. He was as fractious and troublesome as a caged wild beast, which in effect he was. Often during the night he would yell and moan for hours on end, giving the village no rest. On one occasion his parents chained him by the waist to a tree on the outskirts of the settlement. It was a bright moonlit night, and two wolf cubs, who may have been his companions in the den where he was captured, were attracted by the cries they heard from him while prowling, and came down to the tree. They were seen to gambol around him with apparent familiarity and affection as if they recognized him as one of themselves. They left him only when the village stirred at dawn. ¶ This boy did not survive long, and, like the others, he never spoke a recognizable word. An Anglo-Indian civil servant, who had studied many cases and actually seen and examined one recovered wolf-child, wrote the following:

A young she-wolf has a litter of cubs, and after a time her instinct tells her that they will require fresh food. She steals out at night in quest of prey. She espies a weak place in the fence surrounding the compound of a poor villager and penetrates the area, in reality hunting for a kid which she can take home to her cubs. While prowling around she looks into a hut where a woman and child are soundly sleeping. She pounces on the child and is out of reach before its cries can attract the villagers. She gets safely to her den among the rocks and drops the child among her cubs. At this critical moment the fate of the child is in the balance. Either it will immediately be torn to pieces and devoured – or the extreme odds of survival come off. Possibly the cubs are already gorged when the child is thrown before them. Possibly the mother has mis-timed her understanding of what they need, and offered them solid food before they are yet ready for their role as carnivores. If the cubs do not immediately lacerate the child, they will lick it. They will like what they lick, since the baby has been rubbed every day by his own mother with a vegetable oil which Hindu mothers use. The child lies in the nest, getting licked, acquiring the smell of the cubs, and once it has completely assimilated this smell the she-wolf will not molest it. Soon the baby may feel hungry, and hearing the cubs suck the mother it will blindly try to do the same. The she-wolf will even help it. The adoption is complete and the foster-mother will now guard the child like her own flesh and blood. ¶ But the child must soon walk. All wolf-children get along on all fours – but on their elbows and knees, not their hands and knees. Possibly the elbow gives better support to the head and trunk of a young child, or possibly this is the best imitation of wolf-cubs that the imitative child can perform. ¶ Some of these waifs have been recovered after spending ten or more years in the company of wolves. They have a short life ahead of them, and a greatly disturbed one. They are wild and savage, though in a few months they may become more tractable. They rarely stand upright, except to look around their immediate surroundings. They fear the approach of adults, and will growl and snarl at children, but they will welcome pariah dogs and jackals and even share their food with them. They rarely have time to learn to speak, even if they have the inclination, which has never been really satisfactorily tested. For, although they may have the most robust constitutions when they are recovered, they sicken and die almost without exception, and rarely last two years.

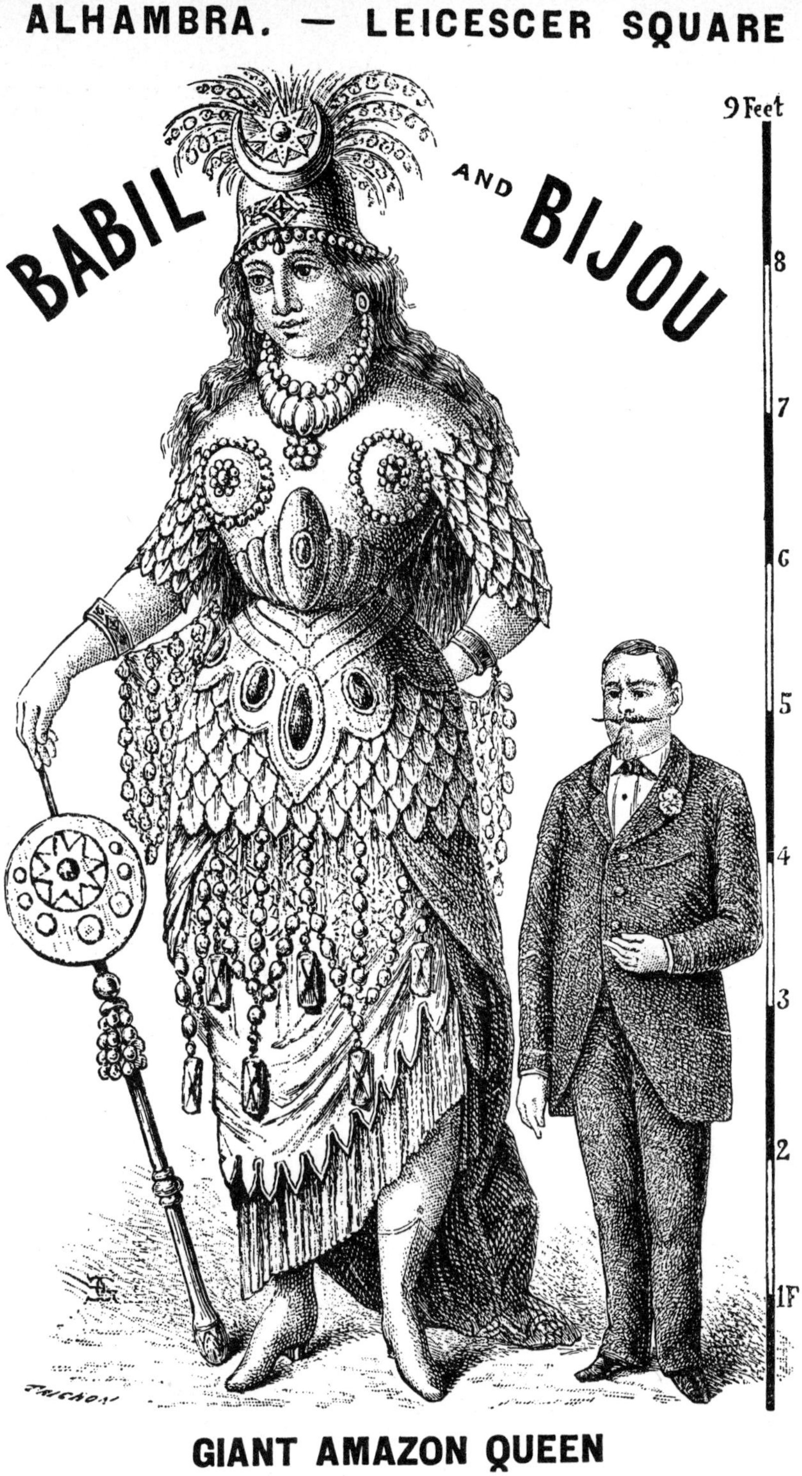

Miss Marian, at a little over 8 feet, was a great success in her review *Babil and Bijou* which played in London in 1882.

CHAPTER SIX

STRANGE CUSTOMS, STRANGER MISFORTUNES

CURIOUSER AND CURIOUSER, the Victorians continued to pry into the unexpected major and minor crises of life. Dr Winn of St Louis reported the case of a man who, when prompted to indulge in sexual intercourse, was immediately prior to the act seized with a fit of sneezing. Even the thought of sexual pleasure with a female was sufficient to provoke this peculiar allergy. ¶ Dr Sullivan of Detroit filed the case of a bride of four weeks, who called at his office saying that in coitus her husband had no difficulty until the point of orgasm, when he was seized with complete numbness and lost all pleasurable sensation in his member. The numbness was followed by a sensation of pain, which was intensified by the slightest motion, and was at times so excruciating that it forbade their separation for upwards of an hour afterwards. The bride asked for advice, but Dr Sullivan had nothing practical to suggest for the immediate relief of the husband's predicament. Sullivan therefore circularized the case throughout the United States medical profession, hoping that some physician would come up with a saving idea. Many doctors gave a distant diagnosis, on the symptoms mentioned. They were all slightly disapproving. The consensus of opinion was that the bridegroom had been in the habit of masturbating and that this exercise had given him a stricture of the membraneous portion of the urethra, which was probably associated with an ulcer of the prostate involving the ejaculatory ducts, or an inflammatory condition of all the tissues compressed by the ejaculatory muscles. None of the doctors could give the bridegroom any instant comfort, however. ¶ Dr Hendrichsen, formerly of Berlin, quoted a case in which, while coitus was proceeding, the woman suffered a spasmodic contraction of the levator ani (the muscle in the pelvis near the rectum which is essential for keeping the guts in position), and the consequent constriction of the vagina was so severe that the penis could not be withdrawn while this condition lasted. Dr Hendrichsen further stated that he himself had been able to bring on this contraction of the levator ani in the patient by conducting a rectal or a vaginal examination, though without any of the preliminaries of coitus. Other people joined this symposium, adding their own experiences of males being held fast in their mates' vaginas, but nobody volunteered a cure, except for the useful negative advice that pails of water should not be thrown over the couple, since this was as impractical as the same tactics when used in an effort to separate a dog and a bitch. ¶ Could people literally die of grief, joy, pride, fear? What did Drs McClintock, Martini, Swingler, and Vincent say? They all said 'Yes'. The old romances were full of people who died from joy after, for instance, being united after long separation, or discovering that a son believed dead was in reality alive and about to make a visit. The doctors said this was possible, and gave chapter and verse of incidents. According to Galen, death from joy was more common than death caused by any other passion, because the condition of joy was much more dangerous than that of anger. Haller said death from joy was probably caused by the blood being sent with such violence to the brain as to cause apoplexy. There was one case on record in which, after a death from sudden joy, the pericardium (the potential space between the heart and the surrounding membranes which allows change in shape and volume of the heart) was found to be full of blood. ¶ Death from violent laughter was recorded, with a rider that such a death might not occur through the emotion itself but through the extreme convulsion and exertion used in the laughter. However, a medical antiquarian, Saint-Foix, looked up from his researches to remark that the Moravians, a sect of Anabaptists, had such a great horror of bloodshed that if they had to execute one of their condemned brethren they resorted to the method of tickling him to death. ¶ Death from fear was well documented. In Victorian times, though happily not later, a frequent cause of alarm so heightened that it led to death was said to be fear of childbirth, or fear of death in childbirth. A number of instances of this were recorded. J. B. Morgagni also mentioned a woman who died from disappointment after bearing a girl baby when she had been desperately hoping for a boy. ¶ A most dramatic death from fear was quoted by J. C. Warren in *Surgical Pathology and Therapeutics*, published in Philadelphia in 1895. Warren had received the case from Lauder Brunton. The janitor of an American college had made himself so obnoxious to the students that they determined to punish him. They therefore prepared a block and a headsman's axe, and set the block up in a lonely place. Some of them dressed themselves up rather theatrically as judges, and the headsman wore suitable tights and head-mask, and when the 'court' was ready a band of students was sent to bring the janitor before it. The janitor at first reacted as if it were all a joke, but the students assured him that they were in deadly earnest. The man was 'tried' by the court and found guilty. He was told to prepare for immediate death. He looked all round him in the hope that he would discern some sign of smirking somewhere, but every face was grim. The man was blindfolded and made to kneel before the block. He heard the executioner raise the axe. Then, instead of the sharp edge, a wet towel was brought down sharply on the back of his neck. The man's body drooped. The bandage was removed from his eyes.

To the horror and astonishment of the students, the janitor was dead. ¶ Why does lightning not only sometimes kill, but add insult to injury by occasionally stripping the body as it does so? Dr Halton of Philadelphia confirmed a partial stripping in 1869 when he discussed the case of a woman struck by lightning in which he had been able to follow the precise course of the current. The woman had been sitting in an outbuilding when lightning struck and shattered a tree a foot away from the building. The flash went away from the tree 7 feet from the ground, penetrated the wall of the building and struck the woman on the back of the head, at a point where her hair was done up in a knot and fastened by two hairpins. The hair was greatly scorched, and under the knot the skin of the scalp was severely burned. The current crossed to her right ear, where there was a gold ear-ring, passed over her throat and down the left of the breast, leaving a blistered burn 3 inches wide. There was another burn 3 inches wide and 12 inches long leading to the pubis. And a burn on her right knee ran right down to her foot, where the lightning had burst open a strongly sewn gaiter boot. The woman was unconscious, but recovered. ¶ Sir James Paget led a discussion on the 'stripping' quality of lightning at a meeting of the Clinical Society of London in October 1879. In one case he put forward, the clothes were wet and the man's skin was reeking with perspiration. He was stripped of everything he wore, his boots were split up from behind, and even the laces were torn out. The Museum of the Royal College of Surgeons displayed a curious collection of relics of a man struck by lightning on 8 June 1878. He was lopping willows with others in a field near Snave, in Romney Marsh, when a violent rainstorm broke. Three of the men entered a shed nearby but the victim – James Orman – stayed by a willow which was close to the window of the shed. A lightning-stroke entered the door, crossed the shed, and passed out of the window, which it blew like an explosive into the field. The men saw that the tree under which Orman had stood was stripped of its bark. His boots stood close to the foot of the tree – but not James Orman. The man himself was naked on the ground farther away. He had been divested of shirt, jacket, vest, trousers, leather belt with buckles, stout hobnail boots, and a watch and chain. All he had on was the left arm of his flannel vest. His eyebrows and beard were scorched off, and his watch had a hole burnt right through it. The watch-chain was almost completely destroyed. A few remaining links and some fused coins had been thrown a distance away. The explanation for the stripping given by the best brains of the time was that the man's clothes were already sopping wet, the electric current had followed their conduction, the heat on the clothes had made a sudden production of steam, and this by its expansion had torn off the clothing and hurled it away. The inference was, therefore, that a man's great working boots in the 1870s could hold enough water to expand and blow them off his feet. That was no mean stroke of lightning. ¶ How does a sword-swallower work, if he is not juggling, and the sword really penetrates his body? This was a common question in Victorian days, unappreciated now since there are no longer any sword-swallowers. Dr Guyot-Daubés of Paris told explicitly how it was done in 1885, and provided a diagram to illustrate it. With a normal person, merely to touch the back of the throat with a finger or a toothbrush brings on gagging, potential vomiting, nausea, and a considerable hindrance to breathing. But the remarkable sword-swallower must first have an imperviousness to these automatic reactions. He must also learn to adjust his body so that what is curved and bent in normal people becomes a straight line in his own case. Many sword-swallowers allowed visitors to touch the stomach and outline the point of the sabre through the skin, so that any hint of counterfeit or juggling had to be dismissed. The sabre used was usually very blunt and with rounded edges – or if it was sharp a sheath of thin metal had previously been swallowed to guide it home, which could be reckoned a necessary precaution. What happened was as follows: the instrument entered the mouth and pharynx, went down the oesophagus, crossed the cardiac end of the stomach and went as far as the antrum of the pylorus, between the stomach and the duodenum. In their normal state in the adult these organs are not

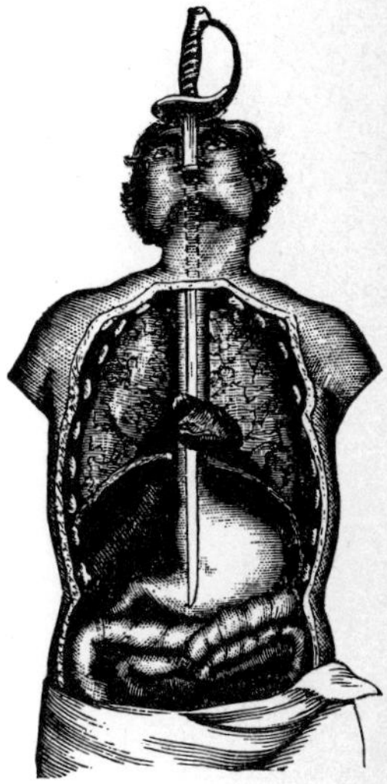

The art of the sword-swallower.

in a straight line, but they were placed so by the passage of the sword. A first essential was that the head was thrown back, so that the mouth was in the direction of the oesophagus (food passage), the curves of which were 'ironed out' as the sword made its entry. The angle made by the oesophagus was obliterated and at the same time the stomach was distended in its vertical direction so that its internal curve disappeared, permitting the blade to traverse the greater diameter of the stomach. Guyot-Daubés calculated that with the average male these organs, in a straight line, extend between 55 and 62 centimetres (about 2 feet), and consequently the performer could swallow a sword of this length. The doctor's divisions of the distance were: mouth and pharynx —10 to 12 cm; oesophagus—25 to 28 cm; distended stomach— 20 to 22 cm. Incidentally, Victorian sword-swallowers were invaluable to the success of one phase of medical research. The Scottish surgeon Stevens was enabled to make his experiments on digestion through the co-operation of a cheerful sword-swallower who took down small metallic tubes pierced with holes which Stevens had previously stuffed with meat, minced and nicely graduated down the tube. After a set length of time the sword-swallower would disgorge the tubes, and Stevens carefully examined the contents. He was thus able to determine the extent of digestion that had taken place at various levels and after varying periods of exposure to the gastric juices. In addition, it was the phenomenon of sword-swallowing which demonstrated to the nineteenth-century physicians the extent to which the pharynx could be persuaded to contract. When they had demonstrated the art of the *possible,* the doctors could then go ahead with much more courage in introducing – as they did in Victoria's day – exploratory tubes for the stomach, methods of washing out the stomach, and even the illumination of the stomach by electric light for telescopic (and periscopic) examination. ¶ Is it possible, is it serious, to fracture the penis? Dr Keen and Dr White explained that the male urethra could occasionally be ruptured during violent coitus, more particularly when employing the reverse of the missionary position, sportingly defined in Victorian

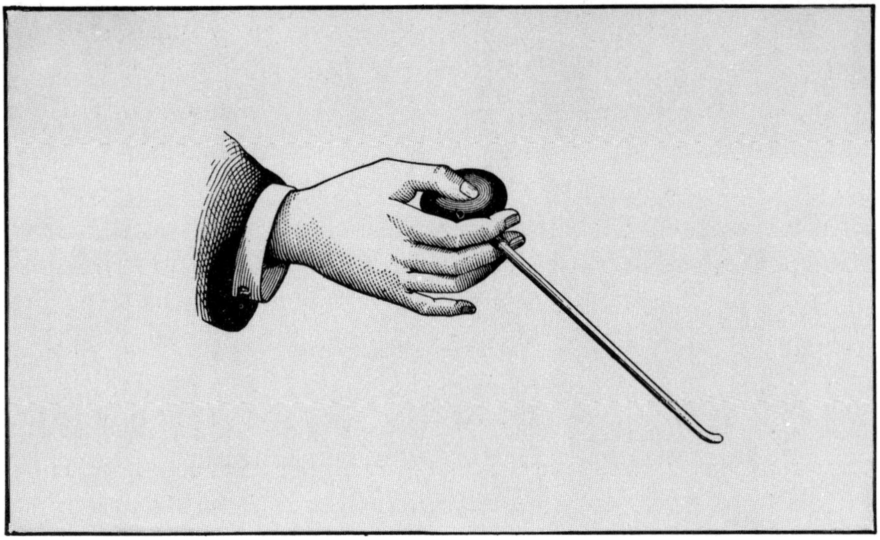

Victorian apparatus for artificial impregnation.

circles as coitus *en postillon*. Watson of Boston gave the grave warning in 1885 that when a patient of his had tried this variation while drunk he had fractured not only the urethra but the invaluable corpus spongiosum into the bargain. Fracture of the penis, which is based on laceration of the corpora cavernosa followed by the extensive extravasation (escape) of blood into the erectile tissue, can sometimes occur during coitus but, Dr Keen whispers darkly aside to Dr White in Philadelphia, has occurred from injury inflicted *accidentally or maliciously*. The warning note about the adverb *maliciously* is that this injury can only be inflicted when the organ is erect. An annoying sequel following this accident, they noted, is the tendency to curvature in erection, which is sometimes so marked as to interfere with coitus, and even render the patient permanently impotent. ¶ An alarming account was available of a twenty-seven-year-old labourer who, in an attempt to urinate with his penis erect, pressed it downwards with such force that he fractured the corpus cavernosum. A further danger, which was more menacing to the Victorians than to their successors owing to the arrival of the automobile age, was that the male member was sometimes amputated by the bite of a furious animal, generally a horse, and often a horse serving in a regiment of artillery – where the beasts seem to have been far more spiteful than in other arms of the service – but sometimes by a donkey and twice, in cases attended by Paullini of Leipzig and Cellier of Paris, by an infuriated dog. ¶ Amputation of the penis was not always followed by the loss of the sexual power and instinct, but sometimes had the effect of temporarily increasing the desire, as Haslam of London reported after attending a deckhand on a whaler who had slipped on the greasy deck and done himself untold damage with his blubber-knife. Haslam had also in his files, which he confided to the *Lancet*, the case of a man who, having entirely lost his penis through circumstances beyond his control, had fashioned for himself a substitute made of ivory. 'Enflamed by the increasing use of this instrument, the fellow finally became so libidinous that it was necessary to exclude him from the workhouse of which he was an inmate.' ¶ Curiouser and curiouser. There was always something to learn for the enquiring Victorian.